PAGE CYCLE DIET

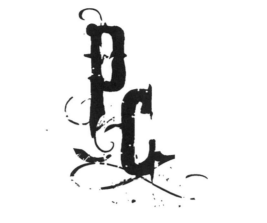

PAGE CYCLE DIET

MIKE PAGE

PAGE CYCLE, LLC

SALT LAKE CITY, UTAH

Disclaimer: This publication contains the opinions and ideas of its author. It is intended to provide helpful and informative material on subjects addressed in the publication. It is sold with the understanding that the author is not engaged in rendering medical, health, or any other kind of personal professional services in the book. The reader should consult his or her medical, health, or any other competent professional before adopting any of the suggestions in this book or drawing inferences from it. The author specifically disclaims all responsibility for any liability, loss, or risk, personal or otherwise, which is incurred as a consequence, directly or indirectly, of the use and application of any of the contents of this book. References are provided for informational purposes only and do not constitute endorsement of any websites or other sources. Readers should be aware that the websites listed in this book may change.

Page Cycle Diet
Page, Mike
Published by: Page Cycle, LLC., Salt Lake City, Utah

Third Edition, Published 2012

Printed in the United States of America

Editor and Interior Design & Layout: Jennifer Du Charme
Cover Art Design: Jennifer R. Phillips, JRP Design

ISBN-13: 978-1466391611
ISBN-10: 1466391618

To the millions who have been
miserable eating to be lean, and to those who have
been miserable eating the foods they love.
That all ends today.

CONTENTS

ONE

You're My Client

I know if you picked up this book, you're seeking a solution to a problem. You're heavier than you would like to be and it's affecting your life in a way that is very personal to you. Whether you want to lose the last 5 - 10 lbs., lose 100 + lbs., or somewhere in between I have the solution for you.

The Page Cycle is a revolutionary "food cycling" program that allows you to see instant results and, more importantly, gives you a long term plan to keep the weight off once and for all. I created this program with over 100,000 hours invested in people just like you who were searching for a way to lose weight (body fat) and keep it off.

The Program has three distinct cycles each designed for a specific purpose…

➢ Cycle 1: Extreme Burn - is designed for rapid fat loss and to get you off to a fast start. The first two days of the plan flip the switch and turn your body into a fat burning machine. Whether you've been programming your body to be a fat storing machine for a month, 6 months, or 40 years, you can literally re-program your body within the first 48 hours.

In just seven days, you'll learn what foods to eat, drop weight and inches, and get on the right track to having the body you have always wanted!

➤ Cycle 2: Burn - is designed for continued fast weight (fat) loss while adding more freedom into the plan. The difference between the Extreme Burn and the Burn Cycle is that you'll be adding more variety of foods in the form of fruits, vegetables, and healthy grains, The other distinction is that you will be adding one free meal each week; that means you get to eat anything you want, with no exceptions, on a weekly basis. Cycle 2 is designed to allow you to "Eat the foods you love, while looking the way you want." By the time you start Cycle 2, your body will be an efficient fat burner while your habits and behaviors will be drastically different.

➤ Cycle 3: Steady Burn - puts you in control of the design of your maintenance plan. I lay all the rules out for you and give you an example of a plan that you can follow (or modify) to suit your personal desires and goals.

Important Notes:

- You can move around within the three cycles to fit your life. If you aren't losing weight fast enough or you gain a few pounds due to a holiday, you can go back to the Extreme Burn cycle and supercharge your results.

Getting to Know You

If we're going to work together, I need to know you better. As you answer these questions, I want you to think of your ideal scenario, and not what you believe is possible. I also want you to dig deep and get emotional with your responses. But first, I want to share a story that has a principle within it that I hope has as big of impact on your life as it had on mine.

Right before I graduated from college, I completed an internship with the only personal trainer I knew of in the Salt Lake area. By the time I finished the internship, I knew personal training was what I wanted to do for a living.

I asked him if he would hire me, and he told me his standard protocol was to have a potential employee fill out a personality profile and have it scored. I did so, but when it came back, I didn't fit his criteria. I was shy and quiet at that period in my life, and that did not fit the profile he was looking for.

I ended up going to work in the physical rehabilitation industry for several years, but I never gave up my dream of being a personal trainer. To make a long story short, I was watching television on Saturday morning when an infomercial came on for Tony Robbins' tape series *Unleash The Power Within*. I immediately bought it. At the end of the first tape, Tony gave an assignment: do something that you have been putting off that would make a big impact in your life. Mine was to call the man who told me I was not cut out to be a personal trainer.

I picked up the phone and the first thing he said was, "I already told you that you don't fit the profile I'm looking for." I told him that I had changed, that I could do it. He reluctantly said to meet him on Monday. When we met, he said one thing to me. "Here's your office. I take x (cut of the profits), the club takes x, and you keep the rest."

I showed up the next morning at 5a.m. with my dream of being a personal trainer right in front of me. There was one small problem. In 1992, most people did not know personal training existed. To make it worse, I didn't have a shirt identifying myself as a trainer. Remember, I told you I was shy and quiet... Now I was suppose to approach people, strike up a conversation, and sell them on working with me.

The first two weeks, I sat in the office and literally almost threw up at the thought of approaching strangers. Tony Robbins got me into this mess, and it's a dang good thing I kept listening to his tape series. Tony taught me that every human behavior is driven by two emotions: pain and pleasure.

The only way I was able to overcome my fear of talking to strangers and realize my dream of becoming a personal trainer was to create more pain in not doing the necessary activities than doing them, I can tell you one thing it wasn't easy, but I went on to master the skill of approaching people so well that, within six months, I was busiest trainer in the gym.

I told you this story for a very specific reason. I've sat down and spoken with thousands of people, and I know that unless and until I break someone's outer shell, when asking questions, I will get their default answer - one that is filled with fear, limited beliefs, and an answer that is safe from future failure.

As you answer these questions, do not simply brush over the surface. Sit in a quiet area and dig deep. Think about your weight, as well as the physical and emotional cost of being heavier than you would like. I know that if you're like most people, you have become very good at suppressing these feelings. I'm asking you to do something that will cause pain. To be honest, I want it to cause you pain!

Don't let the same old emotions and actions hold you back from having the life you deserve. In order to make sure that doesn't happen, you have to create more pain. You need to feel more pain in facing your present than the pain of the emotions holding you back.

I promise it will be worth it. I'm here to give you the tools and the plan to get you the results you desire.

- How long have you been heavier than you would like?
- When was the last time you felt you were at your ideal weight?
- How much weight would you like to lose?
- What size clothing would you like to wear?

- Do you have a time frame in which you would like to achieve your goals?
- What do you feel has kept you from losing the weight and achieving your goals in the past?
- How would you feel about yourself if you were at your ideal weight?

The good news is that no matter how you answered the questions above, I've heard the answer and worked with someone with the same situation as you. I've worked hand in hand with them until they reached their ultimate goal.

I want you to know that your goals are just as important to me as they are to you. I take my job as your Body Transformation Coach very personally. I know from experience that depending on your personality, you may need all the details regarding The Page Cycle or you may just want to jump in and get started immediately.

The book is laid out in a way that will suit your personality. If you need all the details first, take the time to review each section and get comfortable with the science behind the program. If you're ready to get started immediately, skip to the chapter "Before You Get Started" on page 81 and dive in. I know everyone is different, but my preference would be that you take the time to read the book the way it's written. Part of breaking the cycle is doing things differently than you have in the past.

Key To Success

The key to your success and long term results is your commitment to follow the program 100%. The difference in following this program between 100% and 90% is the difference between having the body of your dreams or stacking this program on top of all the other failed diet attempts you've had in the past. Give the plan an extra 10% and it will return 50% greater results...

I love analogies! Do you remember the margin of victory in the men's 100m butterfly at the 2008 Olympics, where Michael Phelps barely beat out Milorad Cavic for his 7th gold medal of the games? .01 second. One one-hundreth of a second! That's the length of a fingernail, if I did the math right ((100m / 50.89 seconds) / 100 − 1.965 centimeters = .774 inches).

What if Michael Phelps had decided, "I've already won six gold medals in this Olympics," and only gave 99% in his final race? He would not have won a seventh gold medal. I am willing to bet that even though he had already won six medals, it would have haunted him for the rest of his life if he hadn't given his all.

Take golf, for instance. From 2000-2006, the average margin of victory at the annual PGA Championships was 1.71 strokes – less than half a stroke per day (the tournament is four days long). Tiny difference, right? Not so when it came to prize money. On average, the winner took home $600,057 more than the 2nd place finisher.

Then there's Formula One racing. For the last ten years, the average difference between 1st and 2nd place at the Indy 500 has been 1.54 seconds. However, the winner took home $1,278,813 while the 2nd place finisher took home $621,321. Six hundred grand is nothing to sneeze at, of course, but that's an awfully big drop in pay for a difference of only 1.54 seconds.

I care about you and your results way too much to not drive this point home. Do not wait for the "perfect" window of time when you don't have a family event or party scheduled. There's always a party, holiday, birthday, family barbeque, date night, etc., etc., etc........

The definition of insanity is "doing the same things over and over again, and expecting a different result." In order to have the body you want, you're going to have to do some things differently. Forget what you have experienced in the past or what you think you know about diet and exercise.

90 Day Challenge

One of the most important things that I used to drive home to a client when we first met, was how important it was for them to give me 90 days of focused effort. Why 90 days? 90 days is long enough for someone to reach their ultimate goal or to make significant changes that will lead to their ultimate goal. On the flip side, 90 days is short enough that it doesn't seem overwhelming.

I don't know how much weight (body fat) you want to lose, but I'm going to challenge you right here and now to make a 90 day commitment to me and to yourself to pull out all the stops and give it 100%. I promise you it will change your life forever!!!

Here are just a few of the thousands upon thousands of stories from
people who have already experienced The Page Cycle:

"While on the Page Cycle I have lost 19 pounds and a little over 22 inches in just 11 weeks! This is equivalent to four pants sizes for me--a body size I never thought I would see again. As a 38 year-old mother of four, I have tried numerous diets, including joining national weight loss chains, and trying every diet fad. Every time I saw an infomercial on TV advertising a weight loss pill, I would buy it, believing that "it" would finally be the cure to my weight loss. Sadly, nothing worked and if I did lose a little weight, I would quickly gain it back and then some! On the Page Cycle I saw significant results in just a week--which was overwhelmingly gratifying and helped to spur me on. The system is easy, realistic, and I have never felt hungry or deprived. I cannot believe a simple system of learning to eat the right foods (that were in my pantry and refrigerator the whole time), at the right time, in the right combination is the solution to the weight problem I have had for years! By following Mike's system and taking the supplements that he recommends I am a totally new person with more energy, more self-confidence, and a healthier mind and body." - Marla Brady

"I am SO excited about the Page Cycle! After just 60 days, I have lost 20lbs and 14 inches!!! Having just had a baby 8 months ago, this is the BEST Program I've ever done!! I feel great, I'm not hungry, I don't feel deprived!! This is the first time in my life that I DON'T feel like I'm 'dieting'...what a concept! It's a 'way of life' and actually enjoyable!!

As a busy mom with a 3 year old, an 8 month old and running a huge business, It's so refreshing to do a program where I don't have to spend hours at the gym a day to get the results I want! I am SO thankful to have had the opportunity to use the products Mike recommends and having the privilege to learn from Mike Page!! He is one of the most knowledgeable people I have ever met, or worked with!! This Food Cycling is AMAZING!!" - Michelle Barnes

"I am 62 years young and live with my wife in Myrtle Beach SC. When we got married 39 years ago I weighed 165 at 5'9". Over the years I have been very physically active but with age, work and raising a family my eating habits were not always the best. Gaining one or two pounds each year does not sound like a lot but over 39 years it certainly adds up. When I met Mike Page in August of 2011 I weighed 208. Mike was and has been very encouraging explaining that even with the gym schedule and exercise regime I keep, I had to change my eating habits to lose weight. Does he know what he's talking about!! In nine weeks following Mikes cycle eating plan I have lost 22 pounds. I have done every diet out there from Physicians Weight Loss to starvation and NOTHING has been easier to follow. I have not been hungry and even sometimes feel like I am eating too much. If you will follow his plan and eat what he recommends you too can FINALLY be successful with a weight loss program. By the way I WILL be at my wedding day weight in the next couple of months and will keep it off for the rest of my life." - Ronnie Felts

"Hi my name is Nancy Sustersic and these days everyone calls me the CEO of Fun, but that wasn't always the case. I have been one of those people who struggled with my weight for the majority of my life. That extra weight for me has not only been a physical burden but a sore spot in my family life as well. You know how family can be so honest that it hurts to the point of depression. Whenever my Mom would try to HELP me realize how I looked she'd often say, 'Why don't you lose that weight. You know you were so pretty when you were thinner and you were happier too. So come on Nancy'. I'd cry and turn to my husband and say... 'It's Mom and it's for you.' I couldn't even keep talking at that point. I'd think, doesn't she know how much that hurts to hear! My husband was nice, he'd say 'That's okay, you're working on it.'

Awhile back, I was looking at pictures of me playing dolls with my granddaughter Kaity it was a real low point in my life. I remember that day like it was yesterday. We were reading a book called; 'Fancy Nancy' and I sure didn't feel like that gal anymore. You know children notice too when you don't feel good about yourself. Being at that weight didn't help with the Fibromyalgia that I had since a young child either. I lacked energy and could not focus at all. Just ask my husband, I was just plain sad! Despite continued efforts I just couldn't lose weight.

Well Fancy Nancy is back and Coach Mike let her out! Dropping several dress sizes and not dieting anymore has been life changing. I have my self-esteem again. I'm 61 years old and feel 30. This 'Food Cycling' is what my body was missing. I wasn't eating the right foods at the right time. I lacked enough protein to build lean muscle. I could eat 'Mike's way' the rest of my life! His coaching and texts help me to not only remember when to eat but what to eat as well. I'm in control now.

If you could see me NOW: My little black dress shows off how spunky I feel today. My skin has been one of the most noticeable things that people have been remarking about. It's getting all tight and my chins are gone! I love the simplicity of eating real food and still shedding the weight. I'm down 18 ½ pounds and 24 inches in just 9 weeks without struggling or craving sweets or junk. I have my weight, appetite and health under control and my life back. My Mom would be so proud of me too, and Mom.. 'YOU WERE RIGHT!'

Thanks Coach Mike for showing me the way!" - Nancy Sustersic

"As women, we are very blessed to be able to bear children...it's a really cool thing! But what is not so cool is that it wreaks havoc on our bodies. I had an easy time losing the weight after the first three...but the twins??? That weight didn't come off so easy. It felt as if my metabolism had come to a screeching halt. It was time to wake it up!

Words cannot express my satisfaction with the Page Food Cycle Plan. The plan is easy to follow and the results are fast. I saw results within the first few days and my thoughts were:

1. Wow! I'm not hungry at all!
2. When you weigh out your food, it certainly is surprising how much a serving really is.
3. I have tons more energy than I have had in YEARS! Just doing the few things that he suggested before starting the program made a world of difference. I can run up all four flights of stairs at work without stopping and my legs are not on FIRE!"

By the end of the first week, I was down four pounds and 5-3/4"! Absolutely incredible! The second week was a loss of another five pounds and 5"!

I have now completed week eight and my results are amazing! I've lost a total of 24 pounds and 26-1/4"! I've dropped four sizes and I constantly have people telling me that I look great. What's even better is that I feel great!

I have tried other plans through the years and nothing else works as well as Page Food Cycling. It's simple, sustainable and it's a life style change that will truly change your life!" - Kari

.

TWO

$\diamond$

The Beginning

$\diamond$

As early as I can remember I've always been fascinated by the human body. I read every article I could get my hands on. After two years at a junior college on a baseball scholarship, I enrolled at the University of Utah in their Exercise and Sports Science program. By age 22, I had my Bachelor's degree and was a Certified Strength and Conditioning Specialist. I worked for several years right after graduation in the physical rehabilitation industry. I spent the next 20+ years working as personal trainer. In that time, I performed over 50,000 individual appointments while working with over 4,000 individuals, 99% of whom were looking to lose weight and get leaner. The first ten years of my personal training career I was on fire! I was doing 65 one-hour appointments per week, and when I did have a client quit, which was rare, I would get a call or one of my clients would come in and say, "I have someone who wants to work with you". I loved my clients and they loved me... Although I was doing what I love, the road wasn't always easy...

Miserable Eating, To Be Lean

One of the driving forces behind the creation of this program is that food has always been a nemesis for me. When I ate the way I should in order to look the way I wanted, I was absolutely miserable. I had to give up a great deal of the foods that I enjoyed and loved. When people ate those foods around me, it created a lot of challenges for me personally. I got angry because it made it very challenging for me to not give into temptation and eat those same foods.

Miserable, Eating Foods I Loved

On the flip side, when I ate the foods I loved, I didn't look the way I wanted and I was miserable as well. I blamed everyone around me for my lack of discipline and alienated the most important people in my life. I felt like I was doomed to be miserable.

Thousands of Clients: Same Experiences

I started to realize that most of my clients felt exactly the same way and that they experienced the same things. Consequently, they weren't able to make the long term changes they needed to with their diet in order to get the results they wanted. Many of my clients were able to make the short term changes required to see results, but very few were able to keep it up and would eventually gain back the weight they initially lost. Let me clarify just a bit, when I talk about keeping the weight off, I mean forever! I'm always disappointed when I've worked with a client that has gotten into amazing shape, and I run into them even if it's 10-15 years later and they have gained weight back.

When someone used to sit down with me I would tell them, "Okay, you're going to have to follow this program perfectly for the next 3 to 4 weeks. If you don't, you're probably not going to lose much weight and, in fact, don't expect a lot of weight loss in the first month or so since it's going to take that long to get your body into a fat burning mode."

My experience was that most people just couldn't eat clean enough for a long enough period of time to change the way their body responded to food. Consequently, they were unable to get their body into a fat burning mode.

Personally and professionally, I was very frustrated, and actually gave up training for a couple of years. I didn't feel right about taking people's money when they weren't getting the results they were looking for. I also felt that if I couldn't do it, how could I expect other people to?

How It All Came Together

A few years ago, I was introduced to a network marketing company that had created a weight loss system with the tag line, "cheat and eat and lose weight." I desperately wanted to believe that the program would work. While that program was a disappointment, it did get me thinking.

What if I could create a program where:

- People saw really fast results.
- There was long term flexibility so that people really could eat the foods they loved and still look the way they want.
- A program I could live with and others could too.

I started playing around with that concept, using myself and clients as guinea pigs. I started to see that I could enjoy a lot more flexibility in the foods I ate while still looking the way I wanted to. People started to hear about the type of results others were having on my program and it started to explode virally. In a matter of a couple of months, I had over 300 people within a five mile radius of the gym using and sharing the program with their friends, family, and neighbors.

The Solution - The Page Cycle

The solution didn't come easy. I came across this quote from Thomas Edison as he was inventing the light bulb, "I have not failed. I've just found 10,000 ways that won't work," and started to see my seventeen years of failure, both personally and professionally, in a different light. I now know that all of the frustration I experienced over that time led me to create this program that will touch the lives of millions of people who I never would have been able to help before.

Get Your Life Back

I have people all the time tell me, "Thank you for giving me my life back." As one of my own clients, I can personally tell you that I'm extremely happy about the way I look and feel. The program has put me back in charge of my life. If I stumble, I know exactly how to get back on track. I'm not afraid of holidays, vacations, or long weekends, and I have learned to enjoy food in a whole new way.

I feel so much better about my relationship with food. I never feel guilty about what I eat, and if I gain a couple of pounds, I simply know I can use a "mini course correction" over the next couple days and the weight will be gone.

My goal is to help 10 million people lose 100 million pounds. I feel like my struggles with food, combined with my background as a personal trainer, have enabled me to create a solution that millions of people are desperately searching for. Time after time, I get responses from people like, "This program is so easy!," "I'm back at my high school weight," "I'm loving it!," "I've never ever been in this size before even when I was young."

I'm so excited and feel so grateful to have created something that is helping so many people. If you've struggled with your weight, get on this program and share it with everyone you know.

The Physical Cost of Being Overweight

I feel comfortable saying that everyone understands that being overweight takes a toll on their health, just like people realize smoking isn't good for them. Being overweight is a major risk factor for the three major leading causes of death: heart disease, cancer, and stroke. It's estimated that nearly 300,000 premature deaths are caused each year by obesity. The cost of obesity on an annual basis in the U.S. alone is over 150 Billion dollars. I was watching a documentary the other day that said 33.3% of all children born after the year 2000 will have Type 2 diabetes sometime in their life, a disease that hardly existed 20 years ago.

The Emotional Cost of Being Overweight

My entire life I've had a gift of reading people on an emotional level. I've always been able to tell how someone is feeling even when their words say something different. I've sat across from thousands of people who lacked self esteem, avoided emotional contact, lacked physical intimacy in their lives, and showed no signs of life at all because when they looked in the mirror they didn't like what they saw. Don't misunderstand me. I'm not saying that physical appearance is everything and that if you look good, you're happy. I'll get into more detail in the chapter, "Your Relationship With Food" on page 61. What I did find out is that many of the people I worked with used food to make themselves feel better about something in their life. When they looked in the mirror, all they saw were the effects food caused on their body and they were still left with the original problem they were trying to feel better about. On the cover of the book, it says break the cycle, with multiple references to your physical body. Breaking the cycle has as much to do with breaking the emotional issues that are holding you back as it does with breaking your body's fat storing cycle.

The Emotional Definition of Overweight

My definition of being overweight is quite different than most. My definition of being overweight is not a number based on height or weight. I would never pull out a table or graph that says you're overweight based on these particular factors.

My definition of being overweight is based on a person's comfort level. If someone feels overweight, or uncomfortable about their appearance, they're overweight.

I had a woman sit across from me, at 5'7 and 110 lbs., who told me she wanted to lose weight because she hated how her legs looked in a swimsuit and skirt. During the course of our conversation, she nearly came to tears, because I was the first person who didn't tell her she was stupid and that she didn't need to lose weight. In her instance, she didn't need to lose weight. However, she did need to decrease her body fat and increase her lean muscle tissue. Within six weeks she had the body she wanted and felt amazing about herself for the first time in her adult life. We all have different goals about our physical appearance. My job is to help you achieve your goals, whatever they may be.

My Why and Gift To The World

I love what I do! I have a passion for helping people feel better about themselves. For over twenty years, the way I've done that is by changing how somebody looks on the outside. When someone tells me they want to lose weight, what they're usually saying is, "I want to feel different about myself."

When I help someone lose weight I don't just affect them, I affect everyone around them. When a husband and father loses weight, he has the energy to help out around the house and play with his kids. When a wife loses weight, she feels more attractive and the relationship with her husband improves. When a teenage girl loses weight and feels good about how she looks, she's less likely to seek attention for the wrong reasons. In essence, when someone feels better about themselves from the inside out, everything in life is better.

Heather's Story

Heather is a 34 year old woman with three kids: Braxton is two, Carley is five, and Michael is ten years old. She works from home in order to have money for the extras in life that her husband feels are wasteful. Heather has been married for eleven years and, in general, appears to be happy in her marriage.

Her husband is a professional, makes a good salary, and reminds Heather of this on a regular basis. While he doesn't appear controlling, Heather makes sure to get his okay on any financial decisions outside of the usual household stuff.

She lives in a nice suburb 15-20 minutes outside of Salt Lake City, Utah. Heather loves to golf, go camping, scrap book, spend time with family, go shopping, and spend the occasional night out with friends. But deep down, she feels like she spends all of her time being a taxi driver to her three kids. Between soccer practice, dance, and music lessons, she feels like she barely has time to breathe, let alone fit in the activities she really enjoys.

Most of the people who know Heather would say she has a great life, three wonderful kids, and a great husband who does well financially.

The second Heather's head hits the pillow at night all she can think about is the hectic schedule for the next day. A PTA meeting at school, dance at 3, a 5 o'clock soccer game, and a 7:30p.m. meeting at the church. Heather's perfect life does not feel that way to her. She feels overwhelmed with the role of being the perfect wife and mom. She spends 95% of her time taking care of the needs of other people and only 5% on herself.

What Really Happened to Heather

When Heather first got married, she used to spend a lot of time on her appearance. She made sure her hair and makeup were always done and she had something cute to wear. She took pride in her appearance and felt sexy. The truth is, since Heather put on 40 pounds, she filled up her life taking care of other people and left very little time for herself as a protective mechanism.

You see, if Heather was so busy, she had no time for herself and she did not have to deal with the way she really felt about herself. She put on a smile and, to almost everyone around her, appeared to be very happy with her life. She felt guilty and very rarely talked about the fact that deep down inside, she wasn't happy.

Heather lost who she was and covered that up by being a busy mom and wife. She gained weight with her first two pregnancies and justified her weight gain as being "normal." By the third baby, the pressures of life, combined with the fact she no longer felt sexy, made it easy for her to develop an attitude of, "What the heck. I might as well be happy and eat what I want." And that was the final straw.

After that moment, Heather was never the same physically or mentally. She tried every crazy diet program out there with minimal results, and even when she did get some results, they never lasted. In fact, Heather was afraid to ask her husband if she could spend money on anything diet related. She knew exactly what he would say, "That is a waste of money and you won't stick with it anyway. You never do."

Deep down inside, she knew he was right and resented him for it. Heather felt like she didn't have the discipline to stick with it. She felt hopeless and buried herself even deeper in other things in life that made her feel good, like her kids and food.

When someone asked her how much weight she wanted to lose she would say ten pounds. In reality, she would have loved to lose 30-40 and feel like she used to when she first got married. By that time, Heather had lost almost all hope that she would ever feel good about herself or feel sexy again.

Today, after implementing The Page Cycle in her life, Heather is still a great mom and wife. However, she has rediscovered herself and is truly happy -- from the inside out. She enjoys her relationship with her husband more than ever, and her willingness to sacrifice for her kids is out of genuine love, and not to hide how she really feels. Heather's choice to take control of her life not only affected her life but the lives of her husband and three children.

Dave's Story

Meet Dave. He is a 52 year old successful entrepreneur who owns his own business. Dave was introduced to me by his second wife, Stacey, who is 35 years old and in great shape. I had been training Stacey for about six months and knew she was frustrated that all Dave did was work, and when he was home he was too tired to do much else. She also shared with me that three years ago, before they were married, Dave was in good shape and they used to do all sorts of active things together.

When I met Dave, he was reluctant to share his goals with me. As I pressed him, he told me this was really his wife's idea, not his. I learned early on in my training career that if someone was not willing to open up or had a hard edge to them, the best thing to do was to take them onto the gym floor and exhaust them. After about fifteen minutes of butt kicking, I took Dave back into the consultation area and he really opened up.

Dave really did want to get back into shape. He shared with me that he felt overwhelmed by his business and life in general. In the three short years Dave had been married, he had gained 45 pounds and felt like he had aged twenty years. When he met Stacey he was a young 49, but he now felt more like her father than her husband.

I worked through enough of Dave's issues to allow him to get started with me and I knew I would uncover more as time went on. Three weeks into his training, I finally got him to spill the beans regarding the real issue. Dave shared with me that he hid in his work because he felt powerful at work. He felt in control and no one told him what to do.

Dave didn't have to spell it out for me. I knew from working with Stacey that she was an extremely strong woman, used to getting her way. The better shape Stacey got in, the more inadequate Dave felt, and the more time he spent at work.

Dave committed to me that day to start The Page Cycle and follow it religiously for four weeks. The first seven days Dave lost eleven pounds, and by the end of four weeks, Dave had lost almost thirty pounds and looked like a new man.

The big deal was not his physical appearance, even though he did look fantastic. The big deal was how he carried himself, the spark in his eye, and the energy in his voice. For the first time in three years, Dave felt alive!

After we started working together, Dave hired an assistant at work so he could spend more time at home. Stacey was so grateful to me to have her strong energetic husband back. Almost every time I saw Dave from that point on, he would give me a sincere thank you for changing the course of his life.

Sara's Story

Sara is a type A personality and a very strong woman who is in control of everything she does. Sara is a successful real estate agent and the mother of 3 kids. I grew to really respect and appreciate her in so many ways in the 8 months I worked with her on her weight loss journey.

The first time I met Sara I never thought I would work with her for 8 days, let alone 8 months, and I certainly didn't think she would go on to lose 80 lbs. When I first met Sara she had just gained back the 75 lbs. she had lost on the HCG diet plan that only allows you to eat 500 calories a day and she was feeling hopeless.

I explained to her the reason she gained the weight back was because that particular program caused her to lose muscle tissue. I also told her that only eating 500 calories a day for an extended period of time had decreased her metabolism to the point where it was impossible to keep the weight off.

Being overweight made Sara mad and angry inside. When I would push her on things and dig into what was going on emotionally with her she would blow up at me. When I made her do things that made her feel inadequate she would refuse to do them and make excuses.

Over a period of 8 months Sara lost the same 75 lbs. she did on her previous diet with one major difference. On her previous diet Sara was a size 14 at her lowest weight. On the Page Cycle Sara was a size 8, and two years later she still is! The amazing part of the story is that Sara hadn't been a size 8 since she was in 8th grade. She shared with me that her sophomore year of high school she was a size 14. 16 years later when she tried her band outfit on it fell right to the floor.

Every time I see her it makes me smile. She carries herself with genuine confidence now and has a softer side that makes her even more powerful. Sara feels in complete control of her weight and has the confidence she will keep the weight off.

Sara's favorite tool of the Page Cycle is what she actually coined as the "magic eraser". I used to call them mini course corrections until one day when Sara came in after a binge eating weekend and told me, "I just love mini course corrections, they are like a magic eraser for bad eating weekends."

Frank's Story

Frank lost just over 100 lbs. on the Page Cycle in 7 months. When I first met Frank he was one of the grumpiest people I had ever met. He complained about anything and everything! Frank was so heavy through his midsection that he routinely had pedicures because he couldn't reach his toenails to cut them.

I had been training him for about 6 weeks when he told me he had been engaged twice and both times his fiancé was killed. The first one died in a drowning accident while they were on vacation. The second one died in an automobile accident shortly after their engagement. Within 12 months of the death of his second fiancé Frank had put on 120 lbs.

He found comfort in food and his two giant Siamese cats. Frank hadn't been on a date in over 15 years and used his weight as a shield to protect him from being hurt again. He told me he was convinced he was meant to live alone.

Within several months on the Page Cycle Frank looked like a whole new person. Physically he had dropped almost 50 lbs. and was now able to cut his own toenails, although he still got his regular pedicures he had grown to love. The biggest difference was Frank's demeanor. He was happy and even started to chat it up with a few of the ladies at his apartment complex.

Six months after starting the Page Cycle Frank was in a serious relationship with a lady he met out to dinner one night with a friend. What a difference 7 months can make in someone's life. Frank shared with me that there was no way he would have started dating being 100 + lbs. overweight. He had completely given up on life and was using his weight as an excuse.

I have thousands of success stories like these and each one represents multiple lives changed. Whenever someone tells me they want to lose weight, what they're really trying to say is that they want to feel different inside. I love what I do and my mission is to help you feel the way you deserve about yourself.

THREE

What Kind Of Results Can You Expect?

When I developed the Page Cycle, the one thing I knew is that people had to see fast results. I learned from twenty years of experience and working with over 50,000 people, either directly or indirectly, that if people do not see results quickly they will most likely give up.

Let me just say this before we look at results. As a professional, if I had read these results without having seen it with my own eyes (thousands of times), I never would have believed it.

The Page Cycle delivers results faster than any program I have used or seen in the past twenty years. Let's take a look at what you can expect over the next thirty days. Keep in mind that the Page Cycle is a fat loss program, not a weight loss program. The difference is that the results are from fat loss, not muscle tissue. This results in a much bigger difference in appearance.

The first 48 hours – The average person will lose between three and nine pounds in the first 48 hours. How much someone loses depends on multiple factors: How much someone needs to lose, gender, beginning weight, how long someone has been overweight, why someone is overweight, how much lean muscle tissue someone has, recent weight gain recent, what their current diet is like, etc... I will explain in a later chapter how it is possible to lose that much weight in such a short period of time as well as why it is safe.

"I have never been able to lose weight quickly so I wasn't expecting to see much. I was amazed that after only two days on the Page Cycle I was down 6 lbs. and my stomach looked flatter." - Linda Sanchez

"Over the past few months I have had the opportunity to use a fantastic meal replacement that has netted me some great results. In my first 90 days of taking this meal replacement I lost over 23 pounds. These were great results but I felt like by body hit a wall and I needed something more to help continue my weight loss.

A great friend of mine suggested that you and I get in touch and that first call with you produced the information I was looking for to step up my weight loss journey. In my first 48 hours I'm down 4 pounds and 5.4 lbs after 72 hours. The support you have provided for me has been Awesome!!!

The strategies you provide in your book was exactly what not only myself but millions of people are looking for. I'm going to be fifty this year and I'm committed to getting in the best shape of my life!!! " - Ryan (Ryno) Vanderpool

Days 1 through 7 – The average person will lose between five and fifteen pounds. All of the same factors from above apply here as well. One of the most important factors is how closely the program is followed. The difference between following the program 100% and 90% is 50% better results.

"After five kids, I found myself heavier than I had ever been in my life. I was looking for something to help me get back on track. I had tried dozens of programs over twenty years but didn't have much success. During the first seven days on the Page Cycle I lost nine pounds. Nine months later I'm down over 90 pounds and can wear my wedding dress I wore thirty years ago." - Denise Jackson

"For many years I have fought my weight, using some amazing Meal Replacement supplements I had lost 50 lbs but needed a boost to keep going, after starting on the Page Cycle Diet in just 4 days I had lost an amazing 10lbs more and feel great!" - Dale Peake

Days 8 through 14 – The average person will lose seven to fifteen pounds after just fourteen days on the program. As a general rule, someone will lose about half the weight they did in the first seven days. When we look at this time frame, the biggest factor you need to keep in mind is: the more someone has to lose, the bigger their weight loss number will typically be. Other factors are: Why the person is overweight; Are there any medical issues causing someone to be overweight (such as a thyroid condition); Is someone on medications that make it more difficult to lose; And the biggie... how closely is someone following the program. While the first week is all about the scale, the second week is all about inches!

"I started The Page Cycle at 252 lbs. I felt old, tired and out of shape. The first 8 days on the program I lost 18 lbs and could not believe how much energy I felt. I started the program wearing 40's and within three weeks I lost 32 lbs and my 36's fall off if I am not wearing a belt.

The program changed my entire lifestyle. I have changed my eating habits and the foods I desire. I have gained a completely different perspective on my life. I just finished my first 5 k race today and me and my wife were the first couple to finish the race pushing a double stroller.

I am 15 years older than my wife [Meghan] and I now realize I need to be healthy to take care of her and the kids. This program is more than just a weight loss program it is a program designed to create a healthier lifestyle for myself and my family

I love the freedom I have to eat the foods I love, but I have noticed that I naturally choose the foods that turn my body into a fat burning machine. I feel so much better on the program. When I deviate away from it and eat the foods I used to I just don't feel as good.

The Page Cycle is not a diet program as much as a way of life for me and my family. As a family we don't eat fast food and even our kids are making better choices. I can't say enough good things about the impact this program has made on me but my entire family" - Corey Meredith

Days 15 through 21 – The average person will lose between ten to fifteen pounds after three cycles on the program. During this time, the weight loss starts to slow down, but the inches lost are the most dramatic during this time frame. Factors include: is someone repeating the Extreme Burn Cycle; have they moved to the more Burn Cycle, in additional to all of the other factors mentioned above.

"I've never had much success losing weight. I was a size 16 when I graduated from high school and pretty much had given up on the idea of ever being thin. After three weeks on the Page Cycle, I had lost 16 pounds, but more amazing than that I was wearing size 12 pants, which is something I had never done. Six months later, I'm wearing a size 8 and I have to say it has completely changed my life. I actually feel sexy now for the first time in my life." - Kim Wright

"When I started The Page Cycle, I had a long way to go. After an injury to my ankle I was heavier than I had ever been - at 278 lbs. After three weeks, I was amazed that I was able to take off twenty pounds. I'm in control of my appetite for the first time since I can remember. I still have 80 more pounds that I would like to lose, but I feel confident that I can do it. I don't feel hungry and if I fall off the wagon and gain a few lbs. I know I can take them off quickly." - Martha Franks

Days 22 through 28 – The average person will be down ten to twenty pounds after completing their first thirty days on the program. Many people will find they have reached their goals and will move onto the maintenance part of the program. The one issue you may have is that most of the clothes in your closet will not fit and you will have to go shopping. I've found that most people don't really see this as a problem.

"My goal when I started the Page Cycle was to lose fifty pounds, and in the first thirty days I have been able to take off sixteen of them. I have lost sixteen pounds in the past and I hardly noticed a difference. Not this time. I am wearing clothes that I thought I would need to lose at least fifty pounds to be in. I have learned not to worry about the scale; that it's all about my body fat! I can't wait to see what I look and feel like after the next thirty days on the program." - Sue Jarvis

"When I started The Page Cycle I was 156 lbs and was in a size 10/12. After just three weeks on the program I was able to lose 12 lbs and am back in my size 6's. Not only was I never hungry I felt completely satisfied. The fact that I was eating real food that I enjoyed and that I liked made the plan very simple to incorporate into my life.

I was amazed how much energy I had on the program. I was worried that, because I was lowering my carbohydrate intake that I wouldn't be able to work full time and be a full time parent. I could not have been more wrong. Not only was I able to work full time I started running after just one day on the program and today I ran my first 5k.

I started the program with my husband [Corey]. We had so much fun planning our meals and snacks together which made it easy. I never thought it would be so easy and that it would change the way the entire family eats.

In the past, I have struggled to stick to any diet program longer than a couple of weeks. The fact that I can eat the foods I love on a regular basis makes the Page Cycle by far the easiest program I have ever done.

I don't feel like the Page Cycle is a diet I feel like it is a lifestyle that I can continue for the rest of my life." - Meghan Meredith

I will end this chapter by saying that the only reason I use weight loss numbers is to show that the results on the Page Cycle are very rapid. The last ten years, I trained people in the gym. My main focus, when it came to results, were how people's clothes were fitting. It is possible to lose weight on the scale and be fatter than before. The only way your clothes fit better is if you're losing body fat. Don't get obsessed with the scale; it's only one tool to determine results and, really, is the least reliable. When you run into an old friend and catch up, do you suppose they are thinking, "I bet you Sue is about 180 pounds," or do you think they are saying, "Holy cow, Sue looks amazing." Nobody cares what you weigh! Why do you?

Personally, I check my weight all the time and, honestly, I do not care what it says. I check it out of curiosity more than anything. There are times when I look in the mirror and know that I need to lose body fat, but when I step on the scale my weight is down. Other times I look in the mirror and think, I look really lean, but the scale says I'm up five pounds. I advise you to weigh yourself out of curiosity more than to determine results. Your clothes and the mirror should do all the talking!!!

FOUR

∞∞∞∞∞∞∞∞∞∞∞∞∞∞∞∞∞∞∞∞∞∞∞∞∞∞∞∞∞∞∞∞∞∞∞∞∞∞

The Key To Fast, Effective Weight Loss

∞∞∞∞∞∞∞∞∞∞∞∞∞∞∞∞∞∞∞∞∞∞∞∞∞∞∞∞∞∞∞∞∞∞∞∞∞∞

How many times have you decided that tomorrow is the day you are going to do something about your weight? You eat well, drag your butt to the gym, and at the end of seven days your weight is exactly the same, or may even be up slightly. If you're like most people, the motivation level drops to zero and you quit. Each time you repeat this cycle with the same result, you start to feel like you're never going to lose weight and it's just a lost cause.

First, let me explain to you why this happens, and then I will give you the key to instant results as well as how to turn your body into a fat burning machine.

Break the Cycle of Insulin Resistance

Ivan Pavlov was a noted Russian physiologist who went on to win the

1904 Nobel Prize for his work studying digestive processes. Ivan noticed that every time his assistants would enter the room to feed the dogs, they would begin to salivate. Salivation, he noted, is a reflexive process. It occurs automatically in response to a specific stimulus; it's not under conscious control.

How does this apply to you and your inability to lose weight? This despite the fact that you're working out and changing the way you eat?

Until now, your dietary habits have conditioned your body to respond in a way that makes your body a very efficient fat storer. We have all heard the old adage, "it's hard for an old dog to learn new tricks." It couldn't be more fitting than when it comes to your body's response to food. Even when you make changes to your diet, your body responds the same way it always has - this makes it almost impossible for you to lose weight.

The medical term for this condition is called insulin resistance. Laura Dolson wrote about insulin resistance. "Insulin resistance is an inability of some of the cells of the body to respond to insulin. It is the beginning of the body not dealing well with sugar (and remember that all carbohydrate breaks down into sugar in our bodies). One of insulin's main jobs is to get certain body cells to "open up" to take in glucose (or, more accurately to store the glucose as fat). Insulin resistance happens when the cells essentially don't open the door when insulin comes knocking. When this happens, the body puts out more insulin to stabilize blood glucose (and so the cells can use the glucose). Over time, this results in a condition called "hyperinsulinemia," or "too much insulin in the blood." Hyperinsulinemia causes other problems, including making it more difficult for the body to use fat for energy."

In layman's terms, insulin resistance is bad. It makes it very difficult to lose weight. When I used to sit down with a client I would tell them that they would have to eat almost perfectly for the next three to four weeks in order to get their body into a fat burning mode. What I was really telling them is that it was going to take that long for their body to break the insulin cycle and start responding differently to food.

Get the Body Into a Fat Burning Mode

The key to breaking the insulin cycle is to deplete all the carbohydrates (glycogen) stored in the liver, muscles, and blood stream, thus forcing the body to burn fat. You accomplish this within the first 24 to 48 hours on the Page Cycle.

The first two days of the Page Cycle are protein-only days, which means you're not taking in any carbohydrates. Through normal body functions and daily activity, your body will burn up the body's glycogen (carbohydrate) reserves, breaking the insulin cycle, and turning your body into a fat burning machine.

What used to take three to four weeks with very little weight loss now takes less than 48 hours!!! Later, I will get into more detail about glycogen depletion and how to use it to change your body into a fat burning machine, but you now know the greatest secret to fast fat loss results.

FIVE

Why Rapid Fat Loss Is Safe & More Effective For Long Term Results

What a difference one word makes. If you read the title above, it says "why rapid fat loss" is not only safe but more effective for long term weight loss.

Since I can remember, every time I've heard "rapid weight loss," whether in print or in the media, it has been portrayed in a very negative light. Doctors and health experts advise against losing more than two pounds per week. Others say that if you lose the weight quickly, you have a greater chance of gaining it back.

The most recent rapid weight loss program to come under fire was Fen-phen. Fen-phen was withdrawn from the U.S. market in 1997 after there were reports of heart valve disease and pulmonary hypertension, including a condition known as cardiac fibrosis. In addition to heart valve disease, the use of fenfluramine has been found to increase the risk of developing Primary Pulmonary Hypertension, or PPH. PPH is a rare disease that causes the progressive narrowing of the blood vessels of the lungs.

The rest of the story, not told in the reports, is that when people were prescribed fen-phen they were also advised to go on a 500 calorie per day diet. Fenfluramine ("fen") triggers the release of serotonin, which creates a feeling of fullness, making it easy to stick to the 500 calorie per day regimen. The problem is that the body starts to eat its own muscle tissue in response to the starvation conditions caused by prolonged intake of so few calories.

In these cases, the body started to break down muscle tissue for energy and attacked people's hearts, which is made up of muscle, in the process. It's true that when rapid weight loss involves starvation, it is not healthy and can lead to damaging health effects.

The Page Cycle is a rapid FAT loss program. The difference is that you're feeding your body and its most important fat loss asset, muscle tissue. At no point in the program are you asked to restrict yourself to 500 calories or take any harmful drugs. The Page Cycle was designed specifically to increase, or at least maintain, your lean muscle tissue and turn your body into a fat burning machine.

The second part of the chapter title is controversial and suggests that if you lose weight quickly, you have a much better chance of keeping it off. After twenty years, there are a lot of things that I can honestly say I don't know, but there are things that I'm sure that I know. I know from practical experience (working with thousands of people) that those individuals who lose weight quickly are definitely more likely to keep it off long term. Just so you don't have to take my word on it, here is evidence to back up what I'm saying.

In one study, over 260 women were placed on a weight loss program, and monitored over eighteen months. The researchers then divided the groups into fast, moderate, and slow weight loss based on the amount of weight lost in the first month. The fast weight loss group was five times more likely to achieve a ten percent loss of their body weight at eighteen months than those in the slow group. Women in the moderate group were nearly three times more likely to reach that milestone than the slow group.

Older studies have found the same thing, except the effects of fast initial weight loss were observed to be better when compared as long as five years.

Astrup, Elfhag, and Rossner's 2000 and 2005 research studies found a similar trend, as numerous analyses of weight loss intervention studies showed that a greater initial weight loss, usually achieved in the first 2-4 weeks of treatment, was associated with a better long-term outcome, as demonstrated by a sustained weight loss 1-5 years later.

Another earlier study showed a similar effect: Those who lost the most weight at 36 weeks were able to maintain a better weight loss two to five years later compared to the slow weight loss group, who had actually regained weight.

Surprisingly, despite all the articles I see in magazines and on the internet about how fast weight loss means you're going to gain the weight back quickly, I was unable to find any scientific research that supports that common belief. It's not true that rapid weight loss leads to poor long term weight maintenance.

My personal opinion is that when people lose weight quickly, the process is seen as easy and motivating, making it more likely for people to continue on the program. My job as a trainer is to motivate people to change their habits and behaviors in order to have a positive impact on their bodies. I can tell you from experience that when you ask someone to give up foods and behaviors they love, and the results are slow and grueling, it's a pretty tough sale. Fast = Success!!!

SIX

Why Most Diets Fail

In my twenty years as a personal trainer, I have utilized, in some form or another, almost every diet program in the marketplace. Remember, I was searching for a solution for myself. I would always try the program first and if I had some success, I would introduce it to my clients. During that process I learned a couple of things that may surprise you.

First, I found at least one golden nugget or trick from every program I tried. Second, every program I tried did produce some results even if it was only for a short period of time. I always kept an open mind and realized that I certainly didn't have all the answers.

I can say with certainty that after all of the trial and error, from the hundreds of different programs I have tried, and the thousands of people I have worked with, I know the following things. I also know why most diets fail.

1) Slow initial results - If you do not get off to a fast start and see

results quickly, you're most likely going to give up and fail in your efforts to lose weight. Conventional wisdom says that rapid weight loss leads to rapid weight regain. A new generation of science, however, shows that slow is not necessarily better.

Shape up the fast way: A 2010 study from the University of Florida suggests that the key to long-term weight loss and maintenance is to lose weight quickly, not gradually. Among 262 obese middle-aged women, fast weight losers were those who shed more than two pounds a week. Compared to more gradual losers, fast weight losers lost more weight overall, maintained their weight loss longer, and were less likely to put weight back on.

I could not agree more with the above study. Within a year of starting my personal training business, I learned that if my clients did not lose a significant amount of weight and see results within the first thirty days, the chances of them continuing were very low.

While other trainers focused on the time spent with their clients at the gym, I focused on their time away from the gym and their diet. I made people accountable by weighing them every time they came to the gym. I made them bring their food journal to every workout, and if they were not seeing results, I would really grill them.

I was a terror, but my clients loved me. I was always the busiest trainer in the gym, because I very rarely ever lost clients. The secret to my success was making sure my clients saw big results in the first thirty days.

Even when my clients gained back some of the weight, if they had originally lost quickly, they had a much different attitude. I noticed they were much more positive and had the confidence that they could do it again. On the flip side, for clients that lost weight slowly over a long period of time, any significant weight gain was devastating. Often times, the slow weight loss clients would give up, feeling like it was too hard and not worth it. Most traditional diets focus on long term changes which is great, but most people get frustrated and give up when the results are slow..

2) If you're not eating foods you enjoy on a regular basis, you may have short term results, but you will most likely fall off the wagon and gain back all the weight you originally lost. In order to be successful long term, your diet has to become natural and simply how you choose to eat.

I'm a firm believer that eating something you enjoy, even in smaller amounts, is much more satisfying than eating more of something you don't like. I believe that the psychological satisfaction of food is equal, if not greater, than the physical satisfaction.

I have found, both personally and with my clients, that eating the foods you love does not lead to overeating when the goal is to lose weight. One of the keys to success of the Page Cycle is that you get to eat the foods you love.

Tanya Zuckerbrot, MS, RD, the author of The F-Factor Diet, has counseled over one thousand patients within her practice. Dr. Zuckerbrot designed a study to understand the physiological satisfaction of food. She measured how different foods affect our desire to eat again, influence how much we think about food, improve our mood and energy level, and satisfy our cravings for sweets.

Dr. Zuckerbrot concluded that "how a food makes us feel is more complex than its nutrient profile alone. When making food choices, people need to think not only about what they are putting in their body with regard to nutrients but also how that food makes them feel, including taste and energy level. Choose foods that keep both your stomach and your head satisfied, and you will find yourself less likely to reach for something else to meet an urge."

Here are just a few short stories from several of my clients who are on the Page Cycle.

"I've never been a dieter in the past and weight worries, fortunately, were not a big issue when I was younger. My weight gain started about 3 years ago after 2 miscarriages and a failed attempt at IVF. I needed to do something before my weight really got out of control. I started a very strict diet limiting my calories to 1200 a day and working out 5-6 times a week. I was successful in losing 10+ pounds, but due to the strictness and low calorie intake, I'd gain it back a month or two later. I was truly a "yo-yo" dieter.

Fast forward to August 29, 2011. I found exactly what I was looking for...a weight loss program that would be healthy and easy to follow..The Page Cycle. The Page Cycle didn't feel like a diet because I could actually eat all the foods that I love and didn't have to worry about counting calories. I learned all about food cycling which was something new to me. The Page Cycle worked well because it's very flexible and taught me how to eat the food I love in the right combinations. It gave me the "freedom" to choose.

Finally, an intelligent and honest approach to long-term weight loss that works! No special foods, diets or other nonsense. Just a program that helped me really understand what was getting in my way, helping figure out what I want, and showing me how to get it. In two months, I've lost 19 pounds and 12 ½ inches." - Stacy Miller

"I have tried to diet in the past with very little success. I found myself cheating and eventually giving up within just a couple of weeks. When I started the Page cycle I was over 400 lbs and looking for a solution. The Page Cycle has been a completely different experience for me. I've lost 58 pounds in just over eight weeks, and I have had a cheat day every Sunday since the second week I started the program. No matter how much I am craving something I know that I can have it on Sunday and eat as much of it as I want. For the first time in my life, I feel like I can finally lose all the weight I want and never gain it back." I'm currently down over 110 lbs... - Jeffery Berg

Let's say you have tremendous willpower and can get past the psychological reasons why most diets fail. Your chances of long term success are still low. Not because you failed, but because your diet plan failed you.

3)   Most programs are based on calorie deprivation, which over an extended period of time causes your metabolism to slow. This makes it harder and harder for you to not only continue to lose weight, but makes it virtually impossible to keep the weight off.

95% of the time when I notice my body fat creeping up it's because I'm not eating enough over a long period of time. When I say I'm not eating enough, I mean I'm not getting enough protein. This causes me to lose muscle tissue and I end up gaining body fat. The scale usually stays about the same, but when I look in the mirror, I don't like what I see.

Recently I was reading an article, How Dieting And Age Affect Your Metabolism. The article explained that, "when you diet, especially at low-calorie levels, you break down muscle mass along with fat to meet your daily calorie needs. With muscle loss comes a reduction in caloric requirements because muscle is an active calorie burner."

When I get someone on The Page Cycle who has hit a plateau, the first thing I ask of them is the detailed report of their food intake. I've found that in the majority of cases, people just aren't eating enough. If you are not eating enough protein and calories, several things happen that are counterproductive to losing weight.

First, we have already talked about the loss of muscle tissue due to a restrictive diet. On average, muscle tissue burns between 35 and 50 calories a day, so even a small reduction in muscle tissue will affect your

Basal Metabolic Rate or BMR. In simple terms, restricted calories leads to muscle loss, which leads to a decreased BMR, which is your body's baseline number of calories burned per day just for survival. Lowering your BMR is exactly what you don't want to do.

Second, when you are on a diet, your body has no idea that you're simply trying to look better in your swimsuit. All it knows is that it is not receiving what it needs. Thus, your body's internal protective mechanism automatically kicks in when you don't eat enough calories. This response is as automatic as the daily functions you don't realize are happening: your heart beating, breathing, blinking of your eyes, etc…

In my experience, the worst things you can do when trying to lose weight or body fat is drastically reduce your calories over a long period of time. I've found that people's bodies become "sticky," making it very difficult to not only lose weight, but even to maintain their current weight

The article, Starvation Protective Mechanism states, "your body uses a brilliant primal survival system that is thought to have evolved over thousands of years as a defense against starvation, and means the body becomes super-efficient at making the most of the calories it does get from food and drink."

You need to understand that the body's reaction to prolonged low calorie diets, and the #1 one reason why diets fail, are related. From a physical sense, you're losing muscle tissue along with fat. Muscle is your number one fat burning asset. Most diets don't specifically focus on retaining, or even gaining, lean muscle tissue as you lose fat.

The body is either in a catabolic (break down of tissue) or anabolic state (building up tissue) at any given time. Significantly decreasing calories and going long periods of time without food causes the body to go into a catabolic state, causing significant muscle loss.

I've already supported the fact that being on a low calorie diet for a prolonged period of time can lead to muscle loss, which then causes a decrease in your body's ability to burn calories.

Let's look at how this happens. Michael R. Eades, M.D.'s blog states, "if you're starving, glucose comes mainly from one place, and that is from the body's protein reservoir." It goes on to say, "thus, a starving person can get a little glucose from the fat that is released from the fat cells, but not nearly enough. The lion's share has to come from muscle that breaks down into amino acids."

When you starve yourself, your body utilizes protein instead of carbohydrates for energy. The problem is that instead of using the protein you're bringing in to repair and regenerate muscle tissue, it's using it as energy. You're defeating your dieting efforts by causing your body to lose its most important fat burning asset, muscle tissue.

The human body has no idea you're simply on a diet. Instead, the body, through complex mechanisms, reacts to the stress and situation it is subjected to. When you drastically reduce your calories, the body senses a famine and goes into protective mode. The interesting thing is that the body will protect its most nutrient packed source of energy, fat, and instead chooses to burn muscle as a fuel source. Remember, less muscle equals increased fat storage. What you think you're doing to lose weight is actually sabotaging the very goal you're after.

My experience has spanned over twenty years and thousands of people, and from this, I have learned that diets fail because people fail to recognize what their weaknesses are, and why they have failed on diets in the past. Typically, I've found that most people will fall into one of the following three categories:

Category 1 – Is the segment of the population that I've had the most interaction with over the past twenty years. The average person in this category wants to lose between 10 and 40 lbs. and is continually working on figuring out how to do it.

These people have lost the same weight over and over again only to gain it back after the program they're on becomes boring, or their motivation slips. I've always enjoyed working with these people because typically they see results quickly and they have the motivation to do the work.

The one component of the puzzle that almost all of these people have is that they don't have quite enough discipline to get the remaining weight off and keep it off, or they simply do not know how to do it. I was one of these people for over 20 years. I would be disciplined enough to get to where I really liked the way I looked. The problem was I just couldn't stick to the plan. I would get bored, or my desire for the wrong foods would get the best of me and keep me from either achieving my goal or maintaining my weight. Once I was off track, it was hard to get back on. Example: Jodie was a client of mine who, for most people's standards, looked good the day she started training with me, but her goal was to look great. She worked hard, got in fantastic shape, and her appearance changed as well, but she was not completely satisfied with the way she looked.

She shared with me that she had been trying to lose the last ten pounds for the past five years. After months of trying to convince her to get on my fat burning system, she gave in and told me she would commit to one month on the program. In eight days, she lost the ten pounds that she had been trying to lose for the last five years. She came into gym excited, and shared with me that, before my program, she had worked out on average of four to five days a week for the past five years without the same success. She could not believe how easy it was!!!

She also shared with me that she had some anxiety that she was going camping three out of the next four weekends, and was worried she would gain the weight back. I told her to enjoy her weekends and come back and do a "mini course correction," which is simply the first two days of the Extreme Burn cycle.

I saw her on Monday morning and she was worried that she had gained 3 pounds over the weekend. I told her to trust me. I didn't see her again until Wednesday, and as she walked closer, I could see she had a huge grin on her face. Not only had she lost the three pounds, but she had actually lost an additional pound! For the next three weekends, the scenario was the same. Each time, she lost all the weight she had gained, plus additional weight. After six weeks on the program, she had lost fifteen pounds total and was the envy of every woman at the gym. In less than thirty days, Jodie had lost more weight than she originally wanted, and learned how to keep it off forever.

The most touching part of this whole story is what she shared with me after her weekend experiences. She told me, "I feel free for the first time in my adult life. When I used to go camping with my family, I would feel so guilty after eating all the junk, and it took the fun out of it for me. I'm so happy now that I can enjoy the weekends with my family, and know that within a few days can be right back to where I was before." I started to cry. I knew exactly how she felt because I used to feel the same way! As I write this sentence, Jodie has kept the weight off for over two years.

Category 2 – This person may or may not work out, but is interested in losing weight and typically has more weight to lose than someone in Category 1. The real issue for this group is that food is a source of comfort, entertainment, and, at the end of the day, most attempts to lose weight fail because food is more important to them than looking the way they desire.

I've always had a slogan, "nothing tastes as good as thin feels," which usually did not go over very well with people within this group. Let's face it. Whether we realize it or not, food is a powerful drug.

Example: The first time I sat down with Stacy S., I told her that she could have an amazing figure, and if she would trust me, I would lead her to where she wanted to go. I trained Stacy three times a week for the next five years, and during that time, she got in better shape and lost some weight.

I always felt like she could do better. I could get her to focus for short periods of time if she had a warm weather vacation coming up or a class reunion to go to. She would come in and tell me, "Okay, this time I'm ready to commit. Can you write me a food plan? I promise I will follow it this time."

After this kept happening, I gave up, and when she would ask me to write her a plan, I would make all sorts of excuses. Soon she would quit asking. Five years into her training, I developed the Page Cycle and asked her to give it a try. Twenty pounds later, Stacy has gone from a size 12 to a size 4, and to this day she couldn't be happier.

I always knew she cheated on her diet and didn't tell me the whole truth when I would ask her about it. Stacy later shared with me that even though she claimed she wanted to lose weight, the way food made her feel was more important to her than how she looked. Now Stacy always tells me that, "she can have her cake and eat it too." When you realize that you don't have to give up the foods you love to look the way you want, a whole new world will open up to you.

Category 3 – Until three years ago, I rarely saw this group of people. This group of people typically has the most weight to lose and has given up. Early in my training career, I got a referral from a friend. When John showed up, he told me he had been overweight most of his adult life, and that he had finally gotten to a place where he was ready to lose weight. We completed our session, he wrote me a check for $600, and we set up a schedule for him to come in three times a week for the next month. On his way home, he stopped, got a large pizza and a super-size meal from McDonald's, and proceeded to eat both of them when he got home.

I never saw John again. When I left a message for him asking how to return his $600 dollars, he never returned my call. In the last three years, I have worked with this segment of the population more than in my previous 17 years. In the past, I never felt like I had a solution for this group. I can honestly say that now that I have a solution, I get tremendous satisfaction from working with this group. I have literally watched people's lives be transformed in a relatively short period of time.

Example: I'm going to talk about a different John here. John started on my the Page Cycle because his sister had great results and she was very concerned about his health.

John started the morning of the first day at 312 pounds. On the morning of the eighth day, John stepped on the scale, and to his amazement, had lost 24 pounds. After 180 days on the program, John had lost a whopping 101 pounds! One year later, he has been able to keep off all the weight he lost and, most impressively, is off seven medications.

While you may not fit perfectly into any of these categories, I bet if you think about it, you can identify with some characteristics of one, or all three, of these categories. It doesn't matter why you're heavier than you would like. If you follow the Page Cycle, you will find the solution and be able to lose the weight you want once and for all.

The Page Cycle is designed to lead to ultimate freedom and a plan you can stick with. I have people from all walks of life, with varying schedules, and every possible reason why they are overweight; they are all enjoying the best results of their lives.

SEVEN

~~~~~~

How The Page Cycle Is Different

~~~~~~

As you now know, I had desperately been searching for a solution for myself and my clients for seventeen years before I finally found the solution. I tried hundreds of different programs and learned one good strategy from most of them. I have worked day in, day out with thousands of people over the course of twenty years, who just like you and me, were searching for a solution to a lifelong problem.

Here's what I didn't do in creating this program:

- I didn't take one principle and create an entire program around it. Most popular diet programs out there take a single principle and make it sound like if you do not follow their program exactly you won't see results.

- Never allow you to binge eat again – I don't know about you, but I know for myself and the thousands of people I have worked with, sometimes you just have to eat until you explode. Every time I do this I find myself asking, "why on earth did I eat like that?," but you know what, when I know that I can "cheat" if I want to, it makes it that much easier to eat properly. In fact, the Page Cycle incorporates a free meal/day into the program where you CAN eat whatever you want. When you overeat, you create mental satisfaction, increase your metabolism, and keep your body from going into a protective mode. When was the last time you were on a diet that encouraged you to overeat, and taught you how to use it to speed up your results?

- Take away the foods you love – If you love Nutella and coffee as much as I do, you understand how ridiculous this is. How on earth are you supposed to follow a program that entirely eliminates the foods you love long term? In my opinion, you might as well be in prison if you cannot enjoy food.

- Create a program that you cannot follow – Most of the new diet programs out there have a different name and different twist on the same old story. It's not rocket science that if you change all the foods you eat and completely change your lifestyle, you will lose weight. The problem is that even while paying me $800 dollars a month to personally guide them, most my clients had a hard time doing what I asked them long term (prior to creating the Page Cycle).

Here is what I did do, and what sets the Page Cycle apart from any other program on the market.

- Fast, Fast, Fast results – I designed this program with speed in mind!!! You already learned that the faster you lose the weight, the greater likelihood that you will keep it off. Nothing is more motivating than seeing fast results.

- You get to eat the foods you love – the Page Cycle was designed to allow you to eat the foods you love on a regular basis and the plan leads to long term freedom. The program has a cheat meal/ day built into it every week to allow you to eat anything you want. I designed it specifically so that no foods are off limit. I have a client who has lost over forty pounds, and has eaten at a Las Vegas buffet every week since he started.

- I took bits and pieces of the best programs over the last twenty years and combined them to create the Page Cycle. One program does not typically fit for everyone. By combining the best of everything, along with my own theories, I created a program that virtually everyone can have success on.

- I allow you to binge – periods of increased calories is a valuable tool for increasing metabolism, and, when followed up by periods of decreased calories, becomes a valuable weight loss tool. What this means to you is that you get to overeat and not feel guilty about it. Can you name the last diet you were on that encouraged you to overeat?

- I designed the program to increase or, at the very least, maintain your lean muscle tissue. Muscle tissue is your body's number one fat burning asset. I already explained in the chapter Why Diets Fail that the number one reason for failure is muscle loss. The Page Cycle is a rapid fat loss program, not just weight loss. The end result is that you get to wear the clothes in the size you have always wanted.

- No program has a strategy like the "mini-course correction," which allows you, within two days, to magically erase bad eating weekends and holidays and get your weight loss back on track. The mini-course correction is the first two days of the Extreme Burn cycle and is the most effective strategy, in twenty years, that I have seen to keep your weight loss on track.

The Page Cycle can do the things other programs cannot because it's the only diet program on the market that utilizes a modified concept used by body builders for decades called "carb-cycling." Bodybuilders use carb cycling to get the last remaining fat off their bodies and get their bodies into contest shape.

Now I know what you're thinking. You're not a bodybuilder and have no desire to be one. But I, too, have no desire to be a bodybuilder, and the 30,000 plus people utilizing the Page Cycle did not want to be bodybuilders either.

Let's take a look at why this concept intrigued me and led me to adapt the concept of carb cycling into a program (food cycling) that everyone could use to achieve their weight loss goal, and enjoy the process while doing it.

Let's take a look at the original concept of carb cycling and why it is a preferred method for bodybuilders as they prepare to get into contest shape.

In the chapter "Why Most Diets Fail", I told you the primary reason why diets fail is that you lose muscle tissue while you are losing fat. This decreases your metabolism, making it difficult to continue to lose weight and keep it off.

At contest time, a bodybuilder's goal is to be as big and lean as possible. The problem bodybuilders have always faced is that in the pursuit of getting leaner, they would lose valuable muscle tissue in the process. Typically, they would have to choose between staying bigger or looking leaner, but they could not have both.

That is, until Frederick C. Hatfield, Ph. D wrote the book The Zig Zag Diet, and introduced the concept of carb and calorie cycling. Dr. Hatfield, or his more well-known name Dr. Squat (because he was the first man to ever squat over 1000 pounds), is one of the most respected icons in the fitness industry. He is currently the president of the International Science & Sports Association, has written dozens of books, and served as an Olympic advisor to the United States Strength Team. The guy knows his stuff, so when he came out with the Zig Zag Plan, he revolutionized bodybuilding forever. His stance was that:

- You cannot lose fat unless you are on a negative calorie balance diet.
- You cannot gain muscle tissue unless you are on a positive calorie balanced diet.
- You cannot lose fat and gain muscle unless you alternate periods of negative calorie balance with periods of positive calorie balance.

It does not matter if you are trying to lose total body weight, stay at the same total body weight, or gain total body weight. The zigzag rule applies to everyone. All the time.

By cycling carbs and total calories in a systematic way, he solved the problem bodybuilders had been plagued with since the beginning of the sport. It is a commonly held belief in the bodybuilding world that the only way you can gain muscle and lose fat at the same time is by using carb cycling.

Sounds like the perfect program, doesn't it? Losing fat and gaining muscle at the same time was music to my ears. I was excited to put myself on the program and start using it with my clients. Talk about a miserable disappointment!!! I should have taken a clue that every article I read said this program is not for the faint of heart, and only for the most disciplined individuals.

In order to follow the program the way it was designed, I had to calculate the exact ratio of fats, carbohydrates, and protein each day. I had to figure out the exact number of carbohydrates required each day cycling between low, medium, and high days.

Food took on the exact role in my life I had been trying to escape: Weighing each portion and fearing that if I deviated at all I would not see results. I had to look at food as fuel only and, needless to say, I not only made myself miserable, but also the people around me. This program taught me exactly why I could never have been a bodybuilder... But it did give me an idea!!!

I spent most of my adult life looking for a solution that enabled me to "eat the foods I love, while looking the way I want." If you combine traditional carb cycling, that only the most dedicated people (bodybuilders) can follow, with a concept of eating the foods you love while still looking the way you want, you get the Page Cycle.

I took the concept of carb cycling and combined it with my twenty years of personal experiences to create a program where you see immediate results. Not only that, but you get the long term outlook which enables you to keep the weight off, without constant measuring or calorie counting. In a nutshell, I took a complex system that produces great results and made it work for the average person.

"I never had a weight problem until I was in my thirties. Then I had to have a complete hysterectomy. Then within a couple of years I went through a horrible divorce and the combination of those two things really caused my increase in weight. I tried numerous programs which seemed to work for the first couple of weeks but then I would get to a point where I just could not lose weight. It was frustrating and disheartening to say the least. I have always been someone who believed in pursuing a healthy lifestyle so the fact that weight loss eluded me was devastating! Then through a very dear friend I learned about Mike Page and his food cycling program. I had never heard of food cycling but I was committed to giving it a try! WOW! This by far is the best thing I have ever done for myself! First of all it is simple once you understand the importance of balancing your proteins and carbohydrates and drinking water. I have never once felt deprived, it just becomes second nature and with so many choices you can eat the foods you really enjoy. I have lost nearly 25 lbs and 19 inches in just over 9 weeks. For me this is by far the most successful I have ever been on any plan. I have consistently lost weight each week which is also a first for me. Even drinking water has become second nature to me. I feel so blessed to have been offered this gift. For the first time in many years I actually feel like me again!" - Carolyn Stevens

"Mike Page is a true visionary in the weight loss/fat loss industry. His Page Cycle Program is a paradigm shift to weight loss/fat loss. No more patchcs, powders, potions, lotions, pills, bars or wafers. No more calorie counting & fad dieting that doesn't work. He has put together the Real Deal!!

I'm a 51 year old who stays very active, playing sports, raising 2 boys & coaching. I am 6'4" & weighed 218 pounds with 20.3% body fat. With Mike's program I've lost 10 pounds, 3 pant sizes, inches all over & 3.2% body fat in less than 2 months. In addition, I feel great & have a tremendous amount of energy. This is a program that anyone, male or female can do!" - Jeff Weisberg

EIGHT

◊◊◊

Your Relationship With Food

◊◊◊

I'm not a psychologist, and don't claim to have any training in the field of psychology. However, I feel like I have a Ph.D. in weight loss counseling after spending over 100,000 hours working with people who want to lose weight.

I would see my typical client two to three days a week, with the average client training with me for years. When you spend that much time with someone, you are bound to learn more about that person than almost anyone else in their life. To be honest, I think I knew most of my clients better than their spouses did; the secret bank accounts to hide money, the teller at the bank they have the hots for, and the things that happened while they were on vacation.

I can tell you that having forty or fifty relationships like this at a time, my life was never dull. I was, in many cases, the most positive relationship in someone's life. I was always positive and supportive. I never judged no matter what I was told.

The one exception to this rule was their nutrition. When I first started training, I stuck pretty much to the basics and did not get into people's personal lives too deeply. But I quickly found that whether or not people were following my advice had more to do with their relationship with food than anything else.

I've always had a gift of reading people, and nowhere was it better utilized than getting to the real reason as to why people were overweight. After countless conversations with people who failed to lose weight, because they just could not seem to stick to any program, I came to this conclusion: At the end of the day, people associate more pain to changing the way they eat and the feelings associated with food than the way being overweight makes them feel. The saying, "people will do more to avoid pain than to gain pleasure," definitely applies to the average person when it comes to dieting.

I've heard every possible excuse why someone is not able to change their dietary habits. "It's too hard," "what are my kids supposed to eat," (by the way thing you eat, if it's not good for you why would it be good for your kids) "I'm too busy," "I can't give up my 600 calorie mocha coffee in the morning or I might die," "I'm punishing my husband by being fat because he had an affair," "I just don't like healthy food," to "I get so hungry."

What I hear is, "It's not worth it," "I don't care," "my coffee is one thing that is just mine and I'm not giving it up," "I'm afraid of intimacy," "I love the way junk food makes me feel," "I love my relationship with food; it never lets me down."

These are the main associations with food that I have found make it very difficult for people to make the changes they need to in order to lose weight and keep it off.

Food is associated with fun. Throughout the years, I've had quite a few clients who were alcoholics. For alcoholics, everything revolved around alcohol. It didn't matter if they were going boating, camping, fishing, or going to a concert. The most important part of the event was their alcohol so they could get drunk. The funny thing is, most people will read this and think that is sad. But replace the word 'food' with alcohol in the previous sentences; does that sound familiar? Food is just as addictive as alcohol, but we do not recognize it as something bad. In fact, a recent study suggests that, whether eating food or simply craving it, food lovers appear to have neural activity similar to that of substance abusers.

Food is associated with family. Growing up, my mom would always have dessert ready first thing after dinner. My mom passed away when I was eighteen, and for most of my adult life, I wanted dessert after dinner. I finally realized that what I really wanted was the feeling I had when my mom would serve dessert. I wanted to feel the comfort and love I felt when she took care of me. I found that a very high percentage of my clients had similar situations in their life, where the act of overeating was related to a memory of family.

Food is associated with holidays. The first few years I started training, I would get angry during the holidays. I remember clients coming in and telling me how they stayed up all night baking just so they could take cookies to their friends for Christmas. I would chew them out and tell them, "don't you realize the average person gains seven to ten pounds between Thanksgiving and New Years?" They looked at me like I was crazy and confused. I've mellowed out since creating the Page Cycle. The program allows you, with the use of "mini-course corrections," to enjoy the holidays and still look the way you want.

I'm going to give you the same speech I've given to my clients for almost twenty years:

You have to make a decision that your goals, and the body you want, are more important than food. There is always a party, family reunion, birthday, holiday, wedding, church get together, camping trip, boating trip, sporting event, class reunion, or about 9000 other things that revolve around food.

Nothing tastes as good as thin feels. Food creates short term happiness. What you're left with is how you feel about yourself every day. At the end of the day, your body is the only thing that is with you all the time. It doesn't matter how much money you make, what kind of car you drive, or the designer clothes you wear. How you feel about yourself is always there lurking in the background.

I explained to you earlier that food made me miserable most of my adult life. I was either eating the way I needed to in order to look the way I wanted, or I was eating the foods I loved and did not look the way I wanted.

The relationship you have with food is directly affecting how you feel about yourself every second of every day. The short term gratification food gives you is stealing your long term happiness. I know because I lived it every day for most of my life.

The great news is that the solution is in your hands. You can finally create a healthy relationship with food like thousands of others I have worked with.

"First of all I want to thank you so much for being my guide through this awesome program to lose weight and reprogram my body to be a fat burning machine rather than a fat storing machine. I am 46 years old and have been overweight for over 10 years now. Ever since I had my child, I have struggled with weight and the getting back to my pre-pregnancy weight which I just hit on 11-2-11. I am so overwhelmed in gratitude by what your professional direction has done for me and I am hopeful it will do the same for others.

This program has been revolutionary to me in terms of understanding how the body works and how it is always looking for balance. Through this program, I have reprogrammed my body to switch gears from storing fat to burning fat.

Before I started this program I was in a bible study that addressed food issues and I had to ask myself what my motive for losing weight was and the reasons I eat. I uncovered that I had valued food way more than I valued my relationship with the Lord. Food was my idol and so I became very convicted in my heart that I needed to change. I think this is the first step to permanent change.

The second step to change was to replace what I had believed (which was a lie- that food could comfort me in times of stress or boredom or loneliness, etc.) for the Truth of God and to be completely satisfied in Him and Him alone. I had to put food in its proper place in my life.

Now that being said, the third step was this program. This program had all the ingredients of success to discipline me and give the footing and understanding around my body I needed to have success once and for all. It contained reprogramming my habits and reprogramming my mind both of which are essential for any lasting change.

This direction I have been given on a day to day basis via text messages and emails has been pivotal in keeping me focused on eating right. Developing new habits of eating and thinking differently about food are the essential to success. If you change your eating but do not change your thinking it wont work and vise versa if you change your thinking but do not change your eating it wont work. Both have to change.

This program and product compliment one another very well and I have received big results because of them. We have been taught to eat when we are hungry and not eat when we are not and this program does the opposite. Being hungry is a good sign I am burning fat and in the right direction. If I am not hungry I need to eat more often to get hungry and start up that fat burning engine that is asleep inside.

Since being on this program, I have tried different kinds of foods I would not of ever considered before and enjoy it. I realized I was eating in a box and did not even know it. Being committed to this program and product will bring about the permanent changes I have wanted for a long time now and am forever grateful to the Lord, Mike and the Page Cycle for changing my life." - Theresa Vardakis

NINE

Weight Loss Supplements

I absolutely love supplements. I have used supplements both personally and professionally for over twenty years. I'm going to use a couple of analogies to explain the importance of supplements in losing weight and, ultimately, keeping it off forever.

Losing the weight: Today is finally the day you're going to replace that old cracked driveway. To save money, you have decided you're going to tear it out yourself and have someone else pour it. You go to the garage and find a 16 pound sledge hammer. You raise the sledge hammer overhead and slam it down to the concrete as hard as you can. To your shock, there is almost no evidence of your efforts. Mentally you say, "this is going to be a-little tougher than I thought, but I'm going to stick it out and get the job done." After an hour, you are tired and sweaty, and realize you underestimated how long this was going to take. So you decide to work smarter, not harder. You go to your local hardware store and rent a jackhammer. What a difference having the right tool for the job makes! Don't get me wrong. It was still hard work, and there were a few times you wondered if you were going to make it. But at the end of the day, you got the job done. This might not have happened if you had stuck to the sledge hammer. Supplements are equivalent to the jackhammer! Most people's bodies are sluggish, and in order to change them from the fat storing mode to the fat burning mode, they need the boost supplements give.

Keeping it off: Imagine you have a big beautiful back yard, with flower beds around the outside and cement curbing to separate the flower beds from the lawn. You absolutely love your yard and take pride in it always looking in tip top shape. You have a shed full of all the gizmos and gadgets to keep your yard looking beautiful. Automatic sprinklers, a power mower, a gas weed trimmer, rakes and hoes, a push cart that spits out fertilizer to make everything green, etc.

Now imagine that in the middle of the night, someone comes along, breaks all the lines to your sprinkler system, and replaces all of your fancy equipment with a non-motorized push mower, a machete to replace your gas weed trimmer, broken handles with splinters on your rakes and hoes, and left you with a pile of fertilizer on the ground with no way to spread it. It's important to you that your yard stay looking beautiful and you do not have the money to replace the equipment that was taken. If it's really important to you, the equipment that you have will still get the job done; it will just take longer and it certainly will not be as easy.

Supplements will not do the job for you. They do not replace eating properly, but they will certainly make the job easier and quicker. Personally, I have found that people who continue to use supplements, after they have lost the weight they desired, are much more likely to keep the weight off long term. Typically, the first question people ask me when I first introduce supplements to them is, "do I have to take them forever?" I answer them, "only if you want the benefits of increased energy, a boost in metabolism, and the security and piece of mind that you are getting all of the nutrition your body needs." Personally, I will always take supplements on a regular basis, and I advise the people I work with to do the same.

Throughout the years, I've used hundreds of different products. Here are the supplements categories that I've found produce the greatest results. I could write an entire book on just this section, but I am going to keep it simple.

Protein Supplement

Protein is the backbone of the Page Cycle Diet. I've found that most people have a very difficult time getting the required amount of protein without using a protein supplement on a regular basis. Personally, I haven't gone longer than a week in the last 25 years without using one.

Most people are extremely busy these days! The convenience and ease of supplements, or replacing meals or snacks with a protein drink, is invaluable. I love the convenience of having a protein supplement on hand at all times. I also find that the people that I work with have a lot more success if they supplement their plan with protein.

When I first starting using protein supplements, they tasted awful and it was all I could do to choke them down. Now they taste amazing and satisfy sweet craving!!! I'm all about anything that can satisfy and create mental satisfaction, while still providing the proper nutrition.

Here's what science says: An editorial written on the power protein provided a key to obesity prevention. The study assigned nineteen people to the following diet regimen: two weeks of a weight maintenance diet (15% of calories [energy] as protein, 35% fat, and 50% carbohydrate), and two weeks of an isocaloric diet (30% of calories [energy] as protein, 20% as fat, 50% as carbohydrate). They found that the subjects felt more satiated and satisfied with the isocaloric high-protein diet than with the weight maintenance diet. Additionally, the subjects on the high protein diet actually decreased their caloric intake by 441 calories per day, and decreased body weight by 4.9 Kg.

I've talked a lot about eating protein every three to four hours so your body doesn't start to break down muscle tissue. This was quantified in a study that analyzed the relationship between frequency of eating and adiposity (fat). The researchers studied the eating habits of 1000 men and 1000 women, ages 35 to 69. They found that the number of meals was directly relational to the proportion of men overweight as compared to the proportion with normal weight. They discovered that the proportion of people who were overweight tended to decrease as frequency of meals increased from three or fewer to five or more a day. The proportion of men with normal weight also increased with meal frequency. In essence, the more often you eat properly, the more fat you will lose.

Liquid Dextrin (Fibersol) Supplement

Let's continue by discussing fiber. The daily intake requirement for fiber is between 20 and 38 grams of fiber, but the average American only gets 14 grams daily. Fiber is found in fruits and vegetables, whole grains, beans. etc. The issue is that as you increase your fiber intake from these foods, it's tough to keep your body in a fat burning mode. I recommend using a Dextrin (fibersol), as a daily supplement.

Here's what science says: A two-week long study analyzed and evaluated the beneficial effects of a new indigestible dextrin-containing beverage on lipid metabolism within an obesity-related parameters. A double-blind clinical trial was performed with eighteen male adults. Here are the conclusions:

1.   Serum triglycerides levels were significantly lowered in the test group, while the placebo group did not show significant changes.

2. There was a tendency for total serum cholesterol, VLDL, and B-lipoprotein to be lowered in the test group. Those values were not changed in the test group.

3. Body weight and BMI were decreased significantly in the test group within the two-week administration of the test sample. Body fat ratio and waist/hip ratio were also decreased significantly in the test group by the four-week administration of the test sample. Those reductions had significant differences from those in the placebo group.

What this means is that an increase of digestible fiber into your diet equals a decrease in your body fat. Ideally the protein supplement you use would also contain Dextrin (fibersol).

Essential Fatty Acids

Essential fatty acids - Fatty acids are the basis of fats and oils, and, despite popular belief, are necessary for overall health. These fatty acids are termed "essential" because your body cannot manufacture them by itself. EFAs (or essential fatty acids) must come from food or supplemental sources. They are also essential because they're a component of every living cell in the body and are necessary for rebuilding existing cells and the production of new cells. I notice that I'm leaner and more muscular when I use them. I don't forget my fatty acids very often!!! Much of the research I've read talks about Essential Fatty Acids ability to suppress cortisol levels, which is a hormone released during periods of stress that causes increased abdominal fat. I have noticed a big difference personally, and with the people I coach, with regards to the reduction of abdominal fat.

Here's what science says: The current popularity and understanding of the benefits of omega-3 fish oil could just be a drop in the ocean. Now a recent study has shown that taking fish oil supplements, with regular exercise, can assist weight loss.

http://www.weightlossresources.co.uk/healthy_lifestyle/fish-oil-weight-loss.htm

The study by the University of South Australia took 75 overweight and obese people (with other cardiovascular disease risk factors such as hypertension and high cholesterol levels) and split them into four groups. At the first split, half were given doses of tuna fish oil while the others were given the same amount of sunflower oil which contains no omega-3. Both these groups were then split. Half taking no extra exercise while the others completed three 45-minute runs, at 75% of their maximum heart rate, each week. The participants were encouraged not to otherwise change their diet.

After 3 weeks, three of the groups showed little change. However, the group that were given the fish oil and had done the exercise showed a decrease in body fat percentage plus an average 2kg/4.5lb weight loss.

The results seem more impressive given that no other changes to eating habits were made. Also, the exercise 'regime' was not much more than the recommended levels for everyone; not just those trying to lose weight. When combined with a calorie-counted diet and increased exercise, the effects of fish oil on weight loss could prove substantial.

It is believed that omega-3 oil improves the flow of blood to the muscles during exercise and helps to stimulate enzymes which transport fat to where it can be used up for energy.

Omega-3 oil is widely available as a supplement and as an additive in certain foods and drinks. Its popularity has been boosted by previous studies linking omega-3 to: improved brain and memory function, good eye-development and maintenance plus the ability to reduce the risks of Alzheimer's and strokes.

Extended studies are planned to further understand the effects of omega-3 over a longer period and combined with greater exercise. Although taking omega-3 in its natural form (from fish for example) may give the greatest benefits, omega-3 fish oil supplements could be an effective natural weight loss supplement to combine with an exercise program.

Look for products that contain a combination different oils which will contain Omega-3 and Omega-6's fish oil, evening primrose, flaxseed oil, CLA, pumpkin seed oil. By no means is this list exhaustive but will give you a great guideline of what to look for.

Thermogenic/Appetite Suppressant

The entire goal of the Page Cycle is to turn your body into a fat burning machine. A thermogenic supplement is specifically designed to boost energy and increase metabolism. I've found the best products contain L-Theanine, Green tea, caffeine, essential fatty acids, PEA (Phenylethylamine), chromium just to name a few . I recommend using a thermogenic first thing in the morning to set the tone for the day and get your body into a fat burning mode.

When most people think about thermogenics, they think of the original products that contained ephedrine. The products were effective, but for many people there were negative side effects like heart palpitations, nervousness, increased blood pressure, and more. Eventually, the more dangerous were banned from the market.

A brand new class of thermogenics has emerged in recent years to prove more effective without the negative side effects. Like I said I could write a book on its own just within the thermogenic category. To make it simple I'm just going to focus on two great components L-Theanine and Green Tea.

What science says: L-Theanine – Theanine is an amino acid primarily found in green tea.

Effects on the Brain: Theanine has been shown to reduce mental and physical stress, and improves cognition and mood in a synergistic manner with caffeine. L-Theanine has been shown to both reduce the time that it takes a person to fall asleep as well as decrease the number of nighttime awakenings.

Immune System Benefits: L-Theanine may also help boost the body's immune response to infection by enabling the disease-fighting capacity of gamma delta T cells. A 2003 study, published by the Brigham Women's Hospital, included a four-week trial with eleven coffee drinkers and ten tea drinkers, who consumed 600 milliliters of coffee or black tea daily. Blood sample analysis found the production of antibacterial proteins was up to five times higher in the tea drinkers, an indicator of a stronger immune response.

One of the biggest benefits of L-theanine is its ability to lower Cortisol levels which have been tied to increased abdominal fat. So be sure to pour yourself another cup of green tea.

Green Tea

Green tea is one of the healthiest beverages around. In fact, the health benefits of green tea are so potent and numerous that this drink can claim its rightful title as a 'super food.'

Heart health: The antioxidants found abundantly in green tea, called catechins (which are responsible for most of the health benefits associated with green tea consumption), have potent antioxidant properties that protect LDL cholesterol in our blood stream from oxidative damage. This is very important for the health of our major arteries, because LDL cholesterol that falls victim to oxidative damage will stick to the artery walls, developing into a plaque. When this plaque builds, it causes atherosclerosis, a health condition that chokes blood supplies to the heart, and is the #1 cause of heart disease!

Other scientific evidence shows us that green tea helps to keep our blood thin, thus reducing clotting and the risk of heart attacks. Drinking green tea also helps to reduce high blood pressure.

Cancer Prevention: Cancer prevention is another key health benefit of drinking green tea regularly. Studies with animals, test tubes studies, and large prospective studies all provide strong evidence for the anti-cancer effects of green tea. Those who drink green tea daily are, statistically, at less risk of developing many kinds of cancers, such as breast, colon, stomach, and liver cancer. The Japanese, who drink more green tea per person than any other nation, are considerably less likely to develop cancer than those in the USA and the West.

Several studies show that the antioxidant effects of catechins include anti-tumor activity, especially at the DNA level. Catechins can actually protect DNA from oxidative damage that can turn cells cancerous.

Anti-inflammatory effects: Several studies have found that the catechins in green tea produce anti-inflammatory effects for joint pain and allergic responses. If you're suffering with any kind of joint pain, you may find that drinking a few cups of green tea each day could ease the painful symptoms. If green tea is not your favorite, a great alternative is to take green tea extract supplements, which contain the equivalent antioxidant catechin power as drinking three to twelve cups of green tea each day! Additionally, new evidence is showing that green tea catechins deliver an inhibitory effect upon histamine production, possibly helping to reduce the amount of histamine released, lessening allergy symptoms. This suggests that green tea could be a great help to those with asthma, allergies, and other kinds of histamine based inflammatory responses.

Weight loss: Green tea extract is showing no signs of slowing down as a weight loss supplement. Sales of green tea extract increase every year, and it has become more popular than Ephedrine, the controversial weight loss pill. Lots of great research has shown that EGCG extract from green tea produces significant weight loss results.

In a study reported on in the American Journal of Clinical Nutrition, it was found that green tea extract resulted in a significant increase in energy expenditure (a measure of metabolism), plus also had a significant effect on fat oxidation. The researchers indicated that their findings had substantial implications for weight control. A 4% overall increase in 24-hour energy expenditure was attributed to the green tea extract, but the researchers found that the extra expenditure took place during the daytime. This led them to conclude that, since thermogenesis (the body's own rate of burning calories) contributes 8-10% of daily energy expenditure in a typical subject, that this 4% overall increase in energy expenditure due to the green tea actually translated to a much larger 35-43% increase in daytime thermogenesis.

In another study, for a period of twelve weeks, overweight and obese participants were placed on a diet containing the same amount of calories and a supervised exercise program that consisted of 3 x 60 minutes of moderate intensity cardio per week. One group was given a daily beverage containing 625mg of catechins and 39mg of caffeine, while the other group was given a daily beverage containing no catechins and 39mg of caffeine.

At the end of the study, the group given catechins lost a lot more abdominal fat and total body weight than the group given no catechins.

A study published in The American Journal of Clinical Nutrition looked at twelve healthy men who cycled, at a consistent rate, for thirty minutes before and thirty minutes after given a supplement containing either catechin or a placebo.

The results found that those given the catechins displayed a 17%

increase in fat oxidation (fat-burning) rates in comparison with the placebo group!

Nitric Oxide

In 1998, the Nobel Prize in Physiology or Medicine was awarded jointly to Robert F. Furchgott, Louis J. Ignarro, and Ferid Murad "for their discoveries concerning nitric oxide as a signalling molecule in the cardiovascular system."

Benefits of Nitric Oxide – A Closer Look

• Blood Circulation – Nitric oxide regulates blood circulation throughout the body, increases the diameter of blood vessels, and prevents formation of clots. It assists the endothelial cells in controlling and relaxing blood vessels. Nitric oxide supplements can also boost the oxygen levels within your body, reduce blood pressure levels, and keep your heart healthy and functioning optimally.

• Immune System – The Immune cells within our body release nitric oxide to destroy bacteria, viruses, and other harmful foreign elements that can cause an infection. The quality of blood cells in the bone marrow, the immunity-boosting cells, and the muscle cells is enhanced with nitric oxide supplements. Nitric oxide is also known to prevent tumor and cancerous growths within the body's cells.

• Endurance level – Nitric oxide increases the endurance level of the muscle cells, enabling you to lift heavier loads, and perform strenuous activities with ease. This is one of the major reasons why body builders consider nitric oxide supplementation extremely beneficial.

• Increases Alertness – Nitric oxide acts as an intracellular messenger between various cells in the body, including the nerve cells. With adequate amount of nitric oxide present in the body, the communication between nerve cells is faster, leading to quicker responses, and an increase in focus and vigilance.

• Increases Sexual Energy – One of the most popular benefits of nitric oxide is that it stimulates, invigorates, and amplifies the sexual response mechanism within the body. Sensory and mental stimulation causes the nerve cells to release nitric oxide. This causes the penis muscles to relax, allowing blood to flow into the penis and create an erection. The process remains the same for women too, as blood flow increases in their vaginal tissues. This is why loss of libido and lack of sexual energy might easily be treated with nitric oxide supplementation.

• Pain Relief – Nitric oxide supplementation can provide long-term relief from the pain associated with arthritis and joint inflammation. This is because it activates the anti-inflammatory mechanism within the body cells and helps in reducing inflammation.

• Increases Muscle Mass – Nitric oxide supplements widen the blood channels that lead to skeletal muscles, allowing for better blood flow and an increase in the lean muscle mass. With an increase in blood flow, the amount of nutrients available for the muscles is increased, which again contributes toward increasing the muscle size.

• Better Intracellular Communication – Nitric oxide improves the process of communication between various cells in the body, including the nerve and the brain cells. Nitric oxide supplementation is therefore extremely beneficial for enhancing memory, combating learning abilities, and increasing concentration levels. It also aids in treating various disorders, especially insomnia and gastrointestinal ailments.

In addition to all of these benefits, nitric oxide is also a rich source of essential nutrients such as B-sitosterol, ursolic, ghycosides, plant sterols, and anthrquinoidenes. It is also rich in zinc, calcium, potassium, iron and Vitamins A and C.

Nitric oxide supplementation can help everyone, but it is especially beneficial for people over the age of 40. The reason behind this is simple. When you are young, your muscles, body cells, and tissues are also in their prime – quick and efficient at releasing and producing enough nitric oxide to carry out different bodily processes.

However, as you grow older, your muscles become weaker and the response mechanism of your nerve cells drops. It is then that you need nitric oxide supplements to boost your cellular activity, increase muscle mass, enhance strength and stamina, and improve your sexual performance. Look for products containing Arginine, Resveratrol Citrulline Malate which are converted in the body to Nitric Oxide.

Antioxidant/Mineral/Vitamin Supplement

There is plenty of research to support the fact that the foods we eat today don't contain the same nutrients they did fifty years ago. Adding these supplements ensures your body is getting all the nutrition and protection it needs.

The human body is built for survival. When you're in the process of losing weight (body fat), your body needs to feel comfortable or it will go into the dreaded protective mode. The best way to make the body feel comfortable is to make sure it is getting all the nutrients it needs by taking an antioxidant/mineral/vitamin supplement that provides 100% of the body's daily needs. When the human body functions optimally, the body's immune function is elevated, which is a sign the body feels safe, thus making our continued weight loss (fat loss) possible.

One of the keys to an improved immune system is antioxidant protection. Losing weight increases the oxidative stress the body experiences. The most powerful antioxidant. Oxidative damage is involved in many chronic diseases, including those cited as the major causes of death in Western societies, such as cardiovascular disorders and cancer. Antioxidants may prevent these degenerative processes by various mechanisms including the scavenging of free radicals. Intake of antioxidant supplements is associated with preventing oxidative damages.

A Gentle Cleanse

I recommend a cleanse product if you've had issues with regularity in the past or start having issues with constipation. Sometimes when you change your diet and add more protein it takes a-little time to adjust. A gentle cleanse performs two primary functions. First, it detoxifies the system and assists in flushing toxins from the body. Second, it eliminates plaque from the colon wall that prevents your food from being absorbed properly. You can eat the healthiest diet in the world, but it's no help if your body can't absorb the food you're eating due to a build-up of plaque on your colon wall. You will notice that when your body is absorbing nutrients properly, many of your cravings will be eliminated naturally. Personally, I notice a big difference in the bloating in my midsection; I feel leaner and have less cravings. I look for products containing these components: fennel, senna leaf, ginger root, milk thistle seed just to name a few. In situations where immediate relief is needed Milk of Magnesia is a fantastic choice.

Before I developed the Page Cycle Plan, I never realized that a major portion of the population had a tough time with regularity. A cleanse can make a big difference if this is an issue you struggle with.

The bottom line: supplements can't do the work for you. However, supplements can turbo-charge your results!!! I strongly recommend that you go to www.pagecyclediet.com where you can see the supplements I use personally and suggest to anyone that wants to lose body fat permanently.

TEN

~~~~~~

Before You Get Started

~~~~~~

I'm sure you have heard the slogan "people don't plan to fail, they fail to plan." I can't emphasize strongly enough how important this step is. Even the person with the strongest willpower in the world will fail if they do not plan appropriately.

You're going to be adopting new behaviors and habits throughout this process. I'm so fortunate at this point in my life to be able to work from home and have access to my kitchen, making it possible to eat most of my meals at home. Let me clarify. I'm fortunate because, during the day, I have easy access to the fridge and I don't have to pack tupperware with me everywhere I go. However, I actually find it just as easy or easier to eat out.

My life has not always been this easy! I remember when I was training, my schedule was a nightmare. At one point in my career, I was training from 5:00a.m. to 5:00p.m., twelve straight appointments, five days a week, with six appointments starting at 6:00a.m. on Saturdays. I would cook a bunch of chicken breasts on Sundays and pack my lunch every day.

Quite a few times over the years, I would forget to pack my lunch and I don't have to tell you that when you're starving, it makes it really hard to make good choices!

I have a client named Bill who is a very successful real estate agent. I remember when Bill started training with me, he would always find different excuses as to why he was not losing weight, and they were not much different than all of the other excuses I had heard over the years: "I just don't have enough time to eat healthy," "I have to take clients out to lunch almost every day," "I work late, and by the time I get home, I'm starving."

One day, I had enough of his excuses. We had a close relationship where I could finally tell him that enough was enough. I said, "Bill, why don't you just accept the fact that food and all these excuses are way more important to you than losing weight?" He got silent for a while, thinking, and said, "Tell me what I need to do."

I told him to grab a cooler and gave him a list of things to buy. For the next ninety days, Bill packed his cooler every day, and wouldn't you know it, he lost forty pounds. To this day, he is at his ideal weight. Take a look at the excuses you always tell yourself and create a plan to eliminate those excuses from your life.

I have a ton of flight attendants on this program and, let me tell you, I'm not sure anyone has a crazier schedule than they do. Some of them continue to make the same excuses and remain heavier than they say they want to be. Others have achieved the body they have always wanted by eliminating the excuses from their lives.

Before starting, take these action steps:

1. **Take measurements** – Inches lost and how your clothes are fitting are a much better indicator of your progress than weight on a scale. As you gain muscle and lose body fat, you may not see the big weight loss

numbers on the scale you expect, but percentage of body fat is really the true indicator. To track your progress, use the form provided in this section or make your own.

2. Take a 'before picture that reflects what you currently look like. A picture is worth a thousand words. If you're in network marketing and building a business, you will be able to share your transformation with people over and over again. It will also be a reminder to you of your progress since changes in appearance will, at times, be more dramatic than the number on the scale. Please also remember that muscle weighs more than fat, and the pounds you lose during the Page Cycle program are unlike the pounds you have lost on any other program.

How to take 'before' and 'after' photos

- Take your measurements the morning of the photo shoot or the day before. Do not go to the shoot with measurements more than a week old. At the very least, weigh yourself and take measurements of your chest, thigh, waist, and upper arm.

- Pick an uncluttered spot for your photo shoot, either in front of a wall or in front of a door.

- Men: take off your shirt and wear shorts; ladies, wear a sports bra and shorts or a bikini. You want to be able to see your waist, belly, and thighs.

- Take the photo in portrait mode instead of landscape. You will want to see yourself from head to toe, and make sure you are close enough to see some details.

- If you can get someone to take the shots, great! If not, use a timer and a tripod, if you have one. I find that ten seconds is just enough time to get into place.

- Look straight ahead, and smile if you want. But do not cheat by sucking in your gut.

What Shots to Take

Front View: Stand up straight with your feed hip-width apart. Arms are at your side but floating off your hips a bit; you need to be able to see the shape and width of your hips.

Side View: Stand up straight (sensing a pattern here? No slouching!), arms hanging down at your side. Make sure your hands are in the middle of your thigh. You do not want your hand blocking the outline of your thighs or butt.

Back View: Pretty much the same as front view, but with your back to the camera.

After the Photo Shoot

Upload the photos to your computer and place them in a folder marked with the date. I set up my file folder system like this: Weight Loss/Pictures, and I then labeled individual folders by date. If you do not track your measurements anywhere else, create a document listing the date, weight, and your measurements. Take new pictures every thirty days.

3. **Go shopping!** Make sure you have plenty of lean protein sources like deli meat turkey, chicken, fish, tuna fish, beef jerky, Carb Master Yogurt, lean red meat, seafood, etc. You should be eating half your weight in ounces of protein daily, so keep the fridge stocked with lean cuts of protein. You also want to make sure you have plenty of 'smart carbs' in the house for your 'smart meal' days. A shopping list is provided for you in the appendix.

4. **Make sure you have access to water.** You should be drinking half your body weight in ounces daily. Water is crucial to flush out the toxins your body is releasing as you release fat into your system. Water also plays a critical role in the fat burning system, so make sure you're drinking your

recommended water intake daily.

5. Commit before you start to follow the program 100% - Remember, the difference between following this program 100% and 90% is 50% better results. Sounds like a pretty good investment to me.

ELEVEN

<><><><><><><><><><><><><><><><><><><><><><><><><><><><><><><><><><><><><><><><><><><><><>

Cycle 1 - Extreme Burn Cycle

<><><><><><><><><><><><><><><><><><><><><><><><><><><><><><><><><><><><><><><><><><><><><>

Extreme Burn Cycle is designed for rapid fat loss and to get you off to a fast start.

Give the extreme burn cycle seven days and here is what you can expect:

- Lose 5-15 pounds…
- Turn your body into a fat burning machine!
- Sec your waistline shrink…
- Learn how to turn your body into a fat burning machine anytime within 24 hours!

Most people have a sluggish metabolism. Our bodies have forgotten how to burn fat as a fuel source and the only calories our bodies burn are the calories we eat. On days 1 and 2, you're forcing your body into a fat-burning mode by depleting all of the sugars (glycogen) stored in the liver and muscles.

When your body kicks into a fat-burning mode and starts burning fat the way it is supposed to, you will feel great! You will notice fewer spikes and drops in your energy levels! When your body is functioning the way it should be, your body's best source of energy is fat.

Because your body is burning fat, losing five or ten pounds on this system will seem like more than that compared to other programs, because the inches you lose will come from the stored fat around your midsection!

Why Protein-Only Days?

Your body needs protein-only days in order to deplete all of the carbohydrates in the bloodstream, muscle, and liver stored in the form of glycogen. By doing this, you give your body no choice but to burn fat as its primary fuel source.

Protein-only allows the calories to be low without losing any muscle tissue. The protein assists in building and maintaining lean muscle tissue - your most important asset for burning fat.

Due to the fact that most people eat too many calories from carbohydrates, our bodies become insulin-resistant. This means that every time most people eat, their bodies release too much insulin. When insulin is elevated in your system, your body cannot burn fat and, consequently, becomes more efficient at storing fat.

Protein, unlike carbohydrates, does not contain any carbohydrates, so it has very little impact on raising insulin levels in the body. In as little as 48 hours, the body's cycle of releasing too much insulin is broken and the body can return to an optimal state. When in an optimum state, your body's primary fuel source is fat. All it takes is 24 to 48 hours on the Page Cycle to turn your body into a fat-burning machine!!!

What's the significance of eating days?

On eating days, you get to add carbohydrates back into your program with a "Smart Meal" containing 500-600 calories. Choose a healthy meal that is high in protein and complex carbohydrates (smart carbs). On meal days, it's protein-only before and after your smart meal. Any time you get hungry, just grab a protein-only snack.

For dinner, stick with protein only, like chicken, turkey, fish, etc. Eating protein for dinner is a great way to stay lean for life. Whatever carbohydrates are in your system when you go to bed will likely be stored as fat. Eating proteins will help us avoid that.

Protein is very difficult for the body to convert to fat. The body will use protein to repair and regenerate muscle tissue and other cells in your body leaving little, if any, to convert to fat. A general rule is to eat your carbohydrates early in the day so your body has the chance to use them for energy. Stick to protein later in the day and evening.

Even though it is tempting to skimp on the carbohydrates after the fast weight loss experienced on days 1 & 2, you will only be hurting your weight loss efforts in the long run. In general, the majority of your weight loss in the early stages of the program will occur after protein-only days. However, meal days are equally important to your long term goals. Do not skimp on carbs!!!

After approximately 48 hours without carbohydrates, your body goes into starvation mode; it will start preserving fat stores and begin breaking down muscle tissue to use as energy. Always remember, muscle is your most important fat burning asset. The Page Cycle is designed to increase, or at least maintain, your current level of lean muscle tissue.

Sample 500 Calorie "Smart Meal"

For eating days	Calories	Carbs	Fat	Protein
Chicken Breast (4 oz)	165	0	4	31
Lettuce (1 cup)	8	2	0	1
Brown rice (.5 cup)	108	22	1	3
Apple (large)	88	22	0	0
Tomato (2 roma)	70	14	0	2
Cheese (.10 cup)	46	0	4	3
Totals	507	67	9	41

Important Rules:

- Each and every day you should get at least half your body weight in grams of protein. That is the minimum number and if you go over that is okay. For example, if you weight 150 pounds, you need to get at least 75 grams of protein per day. I want to make sure you understand exactly what this means. 1 oz of meat, chicken, fish, turkey, etc... contains 6 grams of protein. To make it even more clear, you don't want to weigh the protein. What you're looking for is the number of grams contained in the protein you're eating. A typical protein drink has 20-25 grams of protein.

- Each and every day, you should get half your body weight in ounces of water. For example, if you weigh 150 pounds, you need to get at least 75 ounces of water per day.

- Commit to follow the program 100%. The results will be drastically different for you and will catapult you to success.

- The only food allowed other than protein during the Extreme Burn Cycle is celery. I have found that celery doesn't affect the results and adds texture and fiber to the program (See the "Smart Protein List").

- For clarification purposes, protein only really means protein and healthy fats, that is why they are lumped together on the charts.

Eating five or six times per day can seem like a lot. You can use a protein supplement for at least two of those meals, one first thing in the morning and one between 1:00p.m. and 3:00p.m. (typically a time of day where your blood sugars and energy levels are low). I find that using a protein supplement the ideal way to increase my energy and decrease cravings. Likewise, anytime the program encourages a snack, you can substitute a protein supplement.

Notice that each and every morning, you will start the day with protein-only or a protein supplement. When you sleep at night, your body breaks down muscle tissue to use as energy. Consequently, your blood sugar and insulin levels will be highest first thing in the morning.

Starting the day with protein stops the breakdown of muscle tissue, lowers your insulin levels, and sets your body up to be a fat burner instead of a fat storer.

You'll also notice that at no time during the Extreme Burn Cycle are you allowed any type of carbohydrates at night. Carbohydrates' primary purpose is immediate energy used for exercise, so unless you are going for a midnight run and plan on burning those carbohydrates, they will get stored as fat.

You'll also notice I'm asking you to eat between 10-30 grams of protein within 30-45 minutes of going to bed. Day or night, when your body goes without protein for more than four hours, your body starts to break down muscle tissue. As crazy as it sounds, many bodybuilders set an alarm four hours after they go to bed so they can wake up and consume protein. But don't worry, I'm not that crazy...

My preference is that you use a protein supplement supplements that contains at least 10 grams of protein. Most of the repair and regeneration within your body takes place while you are sleeping. Having the added benefits of the additional nutrition a protein supplement provides is optimal. If you don't have a protein supplement on hand, or choose not to use one, any protein source from the smart protein list will do.

Extreme Burn Cycle

Use this calendar to manage your success! The Extreme Burn Cycle is the starting cycle of the Page Cycle that reprograms how your body responds to food. The emphasis is eating protein-only for 4 days and adding back in smart carbs of veggies and fruit early in the day, for 3 days to create contrast within the body. Recommended for the first 2-weeks to maximize results. The Extreme Burn Cycle can also be repeated, following the Burn or Steady Burn cycles, anytime you need to get back on track to your goal.

☐ Protein-Only Day　　　P = Protein

■ Protein/"Smart Meal" Day

	1	2	3	4	5	6	7
Breakfast	P	P	P	P	P	P	P
Snack	P	P	P	P	P	P	P
Lunch	P	P	"Smart Meal"	P	P	P	P
Snack	P	P	P	P	"Smart Meal"	P	P
Dinner	P	P	P	P	P	P	"Smart Meal"

My Notes:

My daily protein amount is (minimum 1/2 your body weight in grams):

My daily water intake is (1/2 body weight in ounces):

On black days, have a "Smart Meal" for lunch (A "Smart Meal" is a 500-600 calorie meal with Protein, Vegetables, Smart Carbs and Fruit if you wish). Then have protein the rest of the day.

Supplements will increase your chances of success see www.pagecyclediet.com for more info.

Fill in below:

Smart Protein/Fat Choices:

Chicken, turkey, beef, roast beef, steak, omelets, jerky, salmon, tuna, halibut, tilapia, cod, shrimp, scallops, lobster, crab, oysters, tofu, eggs, Canadian bacon, string cheese, cottage cheese, mozzarella cheese, Laughing Cow Swiss cheese, Kroger Carbmaster yogurt (higher protein than carbs), avocado, nuts and seeds, olives, olive oil, sunflower seed butter, buffalo, flax seed oil, almond butter

Smart Fruit and Vegetable Choices:

Sweet potatoes, zucchini, asparagus, broccoli, brussel sprouts, spinach, mushrooms, onions, romaine/iceberg lettuce, red/green/yellow bell peppers, celery, cauliflower, tomatoes, cucumbers, green beans, onions, artichoke, cabbage, pickles, hot peppers, leeks, rhubarb, V-8, apples, oranges, peaches, tangerines, grapes, grapefruit, cantaloupe, pears, all berries, pineapple, plums, mango, watermelon

Smart Carb Choices:

Brown rice, wild rice, whole grain rice, veggie pasta, egg noodles, whole grain pasta, whole grain bread, whole grain bagel, oatmeal, fiber cereal, whole grain tortillas, whole grain pita bread, rice cakes, boiled oatmeal, legumes/beans (any kind)

My Shopping List:

The First 7 days

Days 1 & 2

The first two days are magic. Whether you've been programming your body to be a fat storage machine for a month, six months or forty years, you can literally re-program your body to be a fat burner in the first 24 to 48 hours.

The first two days are absolutely critical to the success of this program. The first two days are also called "mini course corrections," and/or "the magic eraser." As you progress to the point where you are at your ideal weight, or a place where you feel very comfortable, the first two days of the program will be used to maintain that weight.

The average person will lose three to nine pounds in the first two days alone. You're not losing muscle tissue like you are on most programs. Rather, you're depleting your body of stored glycogen and starting to lose body fat. The more muscle tissue you have, the bigger the loss in these first two days. Men typically lose twice as much weight than women due to this fact.

Realize that you're re-programming your body, and depending how long it has been responding in a certain way, it may take a while for it to function optimally. You may experience a slight decrease in energy until the body becomes efficient at burning body fat as its primary fuel source instead of the daily food from your diet.

Most people feel better than they have in a long time, even on the first day on the program. Not everyone is the same, however, and I wanted to make sure that if you're one of the few that feels tired, now you understand why. As your body is detoxifying, some people will experience a slight headache. Make sure you follow the water suggestions of half your weight in ounces, and note that any of the detox symptoms you might feel (headache, slight nausea, minor flu like symptoms) are short lived.

The body is ridding itself of the bad so that you can take your health and body to a whole new level.

***During the first week, and especially the first two days, of the program, decrease the intensity and duration of any workout by 50%. After the first week, you can resume your workout intensity to normal. In fact, you'll be surprised that, even after one week, you'll actually be able to increase the intensity of your workouts. The body will be functioning optimally, resulting in the body's ability to utilize energy more efficiently, which equates to better workouts.

Day 3

Don't expect to see any weight loss on day 3. When you introduce carbohydrates back into the system, the body will retain the carbohydrates you eat as stored muscle glycogen that were depleted during the first two days. In fact, if you don't gain weight, you're actually losing body fat which is offsetting the carbohydrates being stored in the muscle. You'll be amazed how much food 500-600 calories seems like and how full you will feel.

Day 4

Amazingly enough, you will already be feeling thinner after just 72 hours. By now, you'll be feeling healthier as your body is flushing out the toxins and your body is burning fat the way it is supposed to. Your body will be back in weight loss mode, and when you wake up on day 5, the scale will move downward.

Day 5

Day 5 is a meal day. Depending on how efficient your body is, unlike Day 3, you may wake up the morning of Day 6 lighter. If you do not, though, do not worry. It may be several weeks before your body becomes efficient enough to lose on meal days. The fact that you don't gain weight on meal days means you're still losing body fat. You will be surprised how little food it takes to fill you up, and how your cravings are at a minimum.

Day 6

Is a protein-only day. Your metabolism is flying!!! Your body has now become a fat burning machine after only five days. By now, you will be down three to eight pounds and feeling thinner already.

Day 7

For most, the morning of Day 7 is an exciting day because your clothes are already fitting better. Today is a meal day, and you might find yourself surprised that you're excited to eat a healthy lunch. You will find cravings are at a minimal, if at all, and your energy is through the roof.

The morning of Day 8, you're five to fifteen pounds lighter and on your way to having the body you have always dreamed of.

***I recommend that you start with two Extreme Burn Cycles before moving onto Week 1 of the Burn Cycle. Going back and forth in this fashion is the fastest way to reach your goal. I've found that most people need two cycles to lock their body into a fat burning mode. The Page Cycle is designed to put you in control of your life.

***You can always go back to The Extreme Burn Cycle any time to put your body back onto the fast track. The program is designed to have ultimate flexibility, and allow you to move between the cycles in order to fit your life.

Get set up for success by making a trip to the grocery store and getting some items to help you. Check out the Shopping List in the Appendix section of the book. By no means is this a complete shopping list, but it is a great start! People are always asking me what to eat. I've always told my clients that eating healthy and eating to be lean are two totally different things. For example, the next time you go to the store, pick up a box of granola cereal and compare the nutritional information to a box of Kashi.

1 Cup of:	Granola Cereal	Kashi Go Lean
Calories	374	140
Fat	10.4 grams	1.0 gram
Carbohydrates	65.5 grams	30 grams
Fiber	8 grams	10 grams
Protein	9.4 grams	13 grams

This is just one example of how a single choice in your day between two healthy items can make the difference between eating to be lean or not. Theoretically, if you chose a bowl of granola over a bowl of Kashi every day of the year, you would ingest 234 (the difference in calories above) x 365 days, or 85,410 extra calories per year! Your healthy bowl of granola would cause you to gain 85,410/3,500 calories = 24.4 pounds in just one year. By no means is it as simple as calories in/calories out. The more important thing to realize is that the difference between two choices can significantly impact your results long term.

Take twenty minutes, go to the internet, and search high protein/low calorie meals, cereals, snacks, etc., and find food that you enjoy eating. Replace the high-calorie foods in your diet that have very little nutrients with foods (that you love) that are low in calories and high in nutritional value. Use this valuable resource to find the nutritional value of any food: www.nutritiondata.self.com. Pay particularly close attention to the car-bohydrate content of the foods you choose. When you look at the cereal example above, everything is fairly even. The significant difference is that granola contains over twice as many carbohydrates that Kashi does. Nothing will slow your weight loss results and cause you to gain weight like extra calories from carbohydrates.

One of the things you will notice from the shopping list is that most of the items on the list are in their natural form and are not processed.

TWELVE

Cycle 2 - Burn Cycle

The Burn Cycle is designed for continued fast weight loss while giving you more freedom and variety. By the time you start Cycle 2, your body will be an efficient fat burner and your habits and behaviors will be drastically different.

*** The Burn Cycle should not feel like you're on a diet***

The Burn Cycle is set up exactly the same way the Extreme Burn Cycle is, with these modifications:

1. Day 1- Protein-only day (Same as the Extreme Burn Cycle)
2. Days 2, 4, 6 or protein-only days on the Extreme Burn Cycle are now Protein/Unlimited vegetable days.
3. Days 3, 5, 7 or Smart Meal days on the Extreme Burn Cycle with protein-only the rest of the day are now Smart Meal days with Protein/Unlimited vegetables.
4. You get one free meal per week where you can eat whatever, and as much as, you want.

5. Add 1 piece of fruit on a daily basis except day 1 (optional).

In order to have the body you want, you have to adopt some new habits and behaviors. Changing the habits you've had for a lifetime takes time. By the time you start the Burn Cycle, you will have completed two cycles of Extreme Burn (fourteen days) and will be amazed how your new way of eating seems so natural.

- Continue to get half your body weight in ounces of water and half your body weight in grams of protein per day (Remember: these are minimums, and if you go over, it is okay).

- Take a long term outlook and realize that life will get in the way of the schedule. Do not use life as an excuse; just make adjustments and continue to move forward with the program.

- Realize you will gain some weight after your free days. The process is normal, and the weight you gain is not fat tissue. When you eat extra calories in the form of carbohydrates your body will store them in the muscle as glycogen, which is why you will gain weight. The first time you really overdo it and you gain what seems like a lot of weight, you will probably freak out like most people do. However, when you follow that up with a protein day or two, and you not only lose the weight you gained, but additional pounds as well, you will realize a freedom you never thought was possible.

Days 3, 5, 7 - Smart Meal Days

As you can see, the calendar provided lays out everything in a simple way. I wanted to throw in a couple of sample 500-600 calorie meals just to give you some ideas. Take some time and perform an internet search for high protein, 500-600 calorie meals. You will also find some recipes located in Chapter 12, "Ten Fat Burning Meals" on page 145. Get creative, venture out, and create meals that are satisfying to you. There is no reason to eat the same thing day in, day out, unless you want to.

Day 7 - Free Meal / Day

Free meals / days are designed to serve multiple purposes.

- The increased calories will stimulate your metabolism.
- It gives you a chance to eat anything you have been craving.
- Binging once a week keeps your body from going into protective mode.

A free meal / day means just that: a free day to eat whatever you want. Let me explain the distinction between 'free meal' and 'free day.' I typically recommend that the first several months on the Page Cycle, you do a free meal instead of an entire free day. With that said, you can make the choice when to switch from a free meal to a free day.

In my case, sometimes I hardly eat a thing on my free day. Not because I'm trying not to eat poorly. Sometimes I'm just not hungry. The whole idea behind a free day is to eat differently than you do on a daily basis. Like I said, sometimes I eat a lot, and sometimes I hardly eat at all.

Burn Cycle

The mid-point cycle of the Page Cycle. You will repeat the Burn Cycle for majority of the time until you achieve your goal weight. The Burn Cycle supports further reduction with four days of protein and unlimited vegetables, and three days of adding back in smart carbohydrates from whole grains, and pairing a fruit with a protein for a healthy snack once daily. Fruit and grain should be eaten early in the day. Choose to reward yourself with one guilt free meal, but suggest eating protein-only the following day.

	All Protein Day	P = Protein
	Protein/Vegetable Day	V = Vegetable
	Protein/Vegetable/Grain Day	F = Fruit
	Optional Guilt Free Meal (1 per week; you choose day)	G = Grain

	1	2	3	4	5	6	7
Breakfast	P	P, V	P, V	P, V	P, V	P, V	P, V
Snack	P	P	P, F	P	P, F	P	P, F
Lunch	P	P, V, F	P, V, G	P	P, V, G	P, V, F	P, V, G
Snack	P	P, V	P, V	P, V	P, V	P, V	P, V
Dinner	P	P, V	P, V	P, V	P, V	P, V	P, V

My Notes:

Fill in below:

My daily protein amount is (minimum 1/2 your body weight in grams):

My daily water intake is (1/2 body weight in ounces):

On black days, eat fruit and vegetable by lunch time. Have protein the rest of the day.

Supplements will increase your chances of success see www.page-cyclediet.com for more info.

Smart Protein/Fat Choices:

Chicken, turkey, beef, roast beef, steak, omelets, jerky, salmon, tuna, halibut, tilapia, cod, shrimp, scallops, lobster, crab, oysters, tofu, eggs, Canadian bacon, string cheese, cottage cheese, mozzarella cheese, Laughing Cow Swiss cheese, Kroger Carbmaster yogurt (higher protein than carbs), avocado, nuts and seeds, olives, olive oil, sunflower seed butter, buffalo, flax seed oil, almond butter

Smart Fruit and Vegetable Choices:

Sweet potatoes, zucchini, asparagus, broccoli, brussel sprouts, spinach, mushrooms, onions, romaine/iceberg lettuce, red/green/yellow bell peppers, celery, cauliflower, tomatoes, cucumber, green beans, onions, artichoke, cabbage, pickles, hot peppers, leeks, rhubarb, V-8, apples, oranges, peaches, tangerines, grapes, grapefruit, cantaloupe, pears, all berries, pineapple, plums, mango, watermelon

Smart Carb Choices:

Brown rice, wild rice, whole grain rice, veggie pasta, egg noodles, whole grain pasta, whole grain bread, whole grain bagel, oatmeal, fiber cereal, whole grain tortillas, whole grain pita bread, rice cakes, boiled oatmeal, legumes/beans (any kind)

My Shopping List:

THIRTEEN

Cycle 3 - Steady Burn

Cycle 3 puts you in control of how you want to design your maintenance plan. By this point, you're a pro and know exactly how to keep the weight off. I follow the plan fairly loosely and make adjustments from day to day.

If I have a special event coming up, or feel like my metabolism needs a boost, I will go back to The Extreme Burn Cycle for seven days and return to the maintenance plan when finished. Typically, I eat whatever I want from Friday afternoon through Sunday. You may not be able or want to take this much liberty and maintain your desired weight. You will have to play with the plan to find what works best for you and fits your life the best.

Follow these rules when designing your maintenance plan:

- Incorporate one to two all protein days per week.
- Always follow up a cheat day with a protein-only day.

- In the evening, stick to protein and vegetables for the majority of the time.
- Focus on getting half your body weight in grams of protein and ounces of water per day.
- Go back to The Extreme Burn Cycle at least once every sixty days for a tune-up.
- Set a target weight (I recommend five pounds) where if you hit it, you either do a "mini course correction" (see chapter 15) or a week of Extreme Burn.

You've worked hard to get to your goal. Do not let food get a stronghold on your life again!

I typically eat whatever I want from Friday afternoon through Sunday. I have found this schedule works the best for me with regards to my personality and lifestyle. I love having the freedom on the weekends to enjoy my kids, go to movies and have popcorn, and just not be on a schedule. With all that said, if I know I am going to a movie Saturday night, I will eat primarily protein during the day so that I can eat popcorn later.

I look at it this way... If I gave you a budget of $100 to buy a new outfit, the first thing you find is a pair of shoes that you absolutely love. The only problem is that the shoes, with tax, cost $97. You then have a choice to either get the shoes and wear something you already have, or keep looking.

I approach most days this way when it comes to nutrition. I make adjustments as the day goes on. If I have a high calorie, high carbohydrate meal for lunch, I stick with protein-only for dinner. If I have a special night out planned, I keep my calories and carbohydrates low all day so that I can enjoy my night out.

You can eat all the foods you love, and still look the way you want. However, you can't eat all the foods you love, all the time, without making adjustments, or you will end up gaining back all the weight you have lost.

Let's hear some testimonials from some people who have made it to their goal and how they have used the maintenance plan to keep the weight off.

"When I started the Page Cycle, my goal was to lose those last ten pounds that I had been working on for at least five years. I not only lost the weight I wanted, I lost an additional five and have kept it off now for eighteen months. I continue to follow the program loosely and utilize the "mini-course corrections" any time I have a holiday or a few days of bad eating. I eat all the foods I love and make adjustments daily to keep my body where I want it. The Page Cycle has changed my life. I no longer fear holidays or camping trips with my family." - Sally

"I had been working out hard for years, but I just couldn't seem to lose the extra pounds. I got on The Page Cycle and, in less than two months, I totally transformed my body and lost 24 pounds. I have been in good shape before, but it was so hard and grueling that six months into [working out], I would get burned out and gain a bunch of weight back. The Page Cycle has been so easy with free weekends to eat whatever I want, never being hungry, and best of all, if I do gain a few pounds, I can get rid of them so quickly I don't ever feel overwhelmed. I have kept the weight off with ease for the first time in my life." - Brandon S, South Jordan, Utah.

PAGE CYCLE
break the cycle

Steady Burn Cycle

The Steady Burn Cycle helps you maintain your goal weight as part of a healthy lifestyle. Eating smart proteins with smart carbohydrates is now habit. The Steady Burn Cycle empowers you with more flexibility of how you choose to eat to sustain your goal weight. Fruit and grain should be eaten before 4 pm. Opt to reward yourself with one guilt free meal during the week, but suggest eating all protein the following day.

	1	2	3	4	5	6	7
Breakfast	P	P, V	P, V	P, V	P, V	P, V	P, V
Snack	P	P	P, F	P, F	P	P, F	P, F
Lunch	P	P, V, F	P, V, G	P, V, G	P, V, F	P, V, G	P, V, G
Snack	P	P, V	P, V	P, V	P, V	P, V	P, V
Dinner	P	P, V	P, V	P, V	P, V	P, V	P, V

My Notes:

My daily protein amount is (minimum 1/2 your body-weight in grams):

My daily water intake is (1/2 body weight in ounces):

On black days, eat fruit and vegetable by lunch time. Have protein the rest of the day.

Supplements will increase your chances of success see www.pagecyclediet.com for more info.

Fill in below:

Smart Protein/Fat Choices:

Chicken, turkey, beef, roast beef, steak, omelets, jerky, salmon, tuna, halibut, tilapia, cod, shrimp, scallops, lobster, crab, oysters, tofu, eggs, Canadian bacon, string cheese, cottage cheese, mozzarella cheese, Laughing Cow Swiss cheese, Kroger Carbmaster yogurt (higher protein than carbs), avocado, nuts and seeds, olives, olive oil, sunflower seed butter, buffalo, flax seed oil, almond butter

Smart Fruit and Vegetable Choices:

Sweet potatoes, zucchini, asparagus, broccoli, brussel sprouts, spinach, mushrooms, onions, romaine/iceberg lettuce, red/green/yellow bell peppers, celery, cauliflower, tomatoes, cucumbers, green beans, onions, artichoke, cabbage, pickles, hot peppers, leeks, rhubarb, V-8, apples, oranges, peaches, tangerines, grapes, grapefruit, cantaloupe, pears, all berries, pineapple, plums, mango, watermelon

Smart Carb Choices:

Brown rice, wild rice, whole grain rice, veggie pasta, egg noodles, whole grain pasta, whole grain bread, whole grain bagel, oatmeal, fiber cereal, whole grain tortillas, whole grain pita bread, rice cakes, boiled oatmeal, legumes/beans (any kind)

My Shopping List:

☐ All Protein Day	P = Protein
■ Protein/Vegetable Day	V = Vegetable
▨ Protein/Vegetable/Grain Day	F = Fruit
☐ Optional Guilt Free Meal	G = Grain

© 2011 Page Cycle, LLC.

FOURTEEN

Putting It All Together

Now that you have an understanding of the Page Cycle Diet, I'm sure if you're like most people, you still have some questions. This section will fill in the holes and give you a very clear picture of how to incorporate the Page Cycle Diet into your life and achieve your goals.

No matter what your goals are, here's how I recommend you get started. I want you to start with, and complete, two cycles of the Extreme Burn Cycle, followed by one Burn Cycle. I consider this one full cycle (three weeks) on the plan. I want you to complete two full cycles in this fashion (six weeks) before you make any modifications.

Before I go into the modifications, please know that I have found this is the fastest way for you to reach your goal. As your coach, I would recommend proceeding in this fashion until you reach your goal weight (appearance). As you can see, I put parenthesis around appearance. I did that because your appearance is directly related to your body fat, not your weight on the scale. You may hit your appearance goal and not be at the weight that you thought was ideal. Before you get started on this program, I want to get something out of the way. You WILL have fluctuations from day to day on this program and your weight loss journey will not be a straight line down. At times, your weight will increase during periods of increased carbohydrates, like free meal days or even on smart meal days. Don't get stuck on the scale!!! Realize the increased weight is just fluctuations in how much stored energy (carbohydrates) is in your body. I'm telling you right now, if you let this frustrate you to the point that you quit, you're just looking for an excuse to go back to being your old self. Enjoy your new body, regardless of what the scale says…

Modifications

One thing that I realize is that one size does not fit all. I realize you may struggle with protein-only days. I realize you may be a vegetarian and giving up vegetables every day is not easy. I know that giving up some of the foods you eat daily is not easy at all! Because of this, I'm willing to bend a bit because, after all, one of the best things about the Page Cycle Diet is that it's flexible; anyone can work it into their life. That said, before I give you the short-term modifications, I'm going to challenge you first. Are you having a hard time? Are you making excuses as to why you can't follow the plan as its designed because you're allowing your old self to keep you from having the body you want?

If you can look in the mirror and be honest with yourself and say that you truly feel that modifying the plan will allow you to get better results long term, I'm okay with that. What I'm not okay with is you complaining that the plan "just doesn't work for you" or that "it's just too hard to follow." I would rather have you be 100% accountable and tell people that food is more important to you than looking the way you want.

Here are the modifications

Once you have completed your first full cycle (two weeks of Extreme Burn & one week of Burn), if you feel that modifying the program will allow you to be more compliant, here are your choices. Realize your results may or may not be as fast as if you followed my initial recommendations. With that in mind, I would rather have you modify than quit altogether.

➢ Option 1 – Alternate 1 cycle of Extreme Burn / 1 Cycle of Burn

➢ Option 2 – Alternate 2 Cycles of Burn / 1 Cycle of Extreme Burn

My preference would be that you choose option 1. The only scenario where option 2 is preferable is if you're a vegetarian.

Creating Contrast

One of the most important concepts of the Page Cycle is the concept of contrast. The plan is written with contrast from day to day, and from cycle to cycle. I really need you to understand this concept, so forgive me if it seems like I'm pounding it into your head and becoming repetitive.

Day to day contrast

Extreme Burn Cycle: In this cycle you have protein-only days and smart meal days. When you do protein-only, you force your body to burn fat. Smart meal days are designed to preserve lean muscle tissue and keep your body from going into a protective mode. When you start to blur the lines and don't follow the program, your results will suffer because you take away the contrast. One of the common problems is that people don't eat enough carbs on the smart meal days in attempt to lose weight faster. The result is lack of contrast between the days and their results slow down.

Burn Cycle: In this cycle there is less contrast between day to day. Make sure that on smart meal days, you focus on eating a larger meal at lunch time and that you add healthy grains and starches. If you don't do this, there will be very little contrast. You also get to add a free meal to eat whatever, and as much as, you want. Go big! The extra calories will stimulate your metabolism and make your body feel safe. If you eat a meal that is no different than your smart meal, there is no contrast. I'm relentless on this, so you're probably going to get sick of hearing me say it!

Contrast between cycles

During the Extreme Burn cycle, it is all about fat burning and keeping carbs to a minimum. During the Burn cycle, it is all about adding variety, calories, getting plenty of fiber, and keeping your body from going into a protective mode. Don't expect a lot of scale weight loss on the burn cycle, especially in the early stages of your program. Look at it as the perfect setup for big losses on the Extreme Burn cycles. I know what a lot of you are thinking, "Why don't I just stay on the Extreme Burn cycle the whole time?" You probably answered your own question, though. Contrast, contrast, contrast! The contrast from cycle-to-cycle is equally important as the contrast from day-to-day.

Support on the Page Cycle Diet

It's estimated that 95% of all people who go on a weight-loss plan put the weight back on within three years. Here are the reasons people are not successful, or if they do lose weight, why they gain it back:

1.   There is no way you can lose weight one way and keep it off another. There are a lot of programs out there that there is no way you can keep them up long term. What happens when they deviate and return to normal, you guessed it they gain all the weight back.

2.   Most weight loss plans are based on calorie deprivation. HCG, a popular diet plan right now, advocates daily injections and limiting yourself to 500 calories a day to lose weight. Again, what happens when

people eat more? Same result: they gain all the weight back, plus more.

3. Lack of education. In the time it has taken you to read this book, you became more educated than 95% of the population on how your body responds to food, how to force your body into a fat burning mode, and the truth that diet is the key to the way you look. Imagine if your auto mechanic had the same level of knowledge about your automobile as the average person has about how to lose weight and keep it off. No wonder 98% of people fail at keeping the weight off once they have lost it!

4. Giving up the foods you love. You might be able to give up the foods you love for a week, thirty days, or maybe even ninety, but eventually, if you're not eating food you enjoy, the weight will come back. The Page Cycle does not ask you to give up the foods you love. Instead, the Page Cycle was specifically designed to teach you how to enjoy the foods you love and still look the way you want.

Frequently Asked Questions

Here are some of the most commonly asked questions I've been asked over the last four years from people utilizing the Page Cycle Diet.

Can I have coffee? Yes, yes and yes! Aside from the fact that I would never develop a program where you could not drink coffee, caffeine actually acts as a thermogenic aiding in fat loss. You can't have your 500 calorie coffee filled with sugar anymore if that's your normal routine, but coffee is on the menu. If you're craving the extra large, sugar, and whipped cream version, just save it for a cheat meal!

What kind of cream can I use? The only kind of cream you can't use is a cream that is high in sugar. Do not use skim milk or non-fat creamers because you think they are better. In fact, the extra fat slows down the absorption of the sugars in the milk; this keeps your insulin levels low. Typically, non-fat products contain more sugar than regular. You can also use creams that use artificial sweeteners.

Can I use artificial sweeteners? Artificial sweeteners are a hot topic these days. You read one research article and it makes it sound like artificial sweeteners are the worst thing on the planet. Read another article and it says there is no clear cut evidence to suggest they are bad in any way. I say yes! I know some of you will probably disagree, and to you I say, just don't use them. I personally use them all the time. I'm grateful they exist - they enhance the flavor of so many things I never ate before due to their high sugar content.

Can I drink diet soda? Yes. My preference is that you do not buy a gigantic mug full first thing in the morning and drink it all day. Some research says it has an impact on your insulin levels, while others do not. Practical experience: The only people I see drinking diet sodas are overweight, and, in general, I have found practical experience to be more reliable than clinical research.

Can I use spices? Use as many spices as you want to add flavor. One of the keys to the Page Cycle is to enjoy the food you're eating.

Can I use sauces? You can use any type of sauce you want, even if it contains sugar. Pay attention though, and read the food labels of the sauces you are using. Many times you can find sauces where you like the taste and they have a lot less, or even no, sugar. I love mustard and use it as much as possible because it has zero sugar.

I know that some of you might be confused that on protein-only days I won't let you eat vegetables, but you can have barbeque sauce that contains sugar? To that I say, trust me. Follow the program the way it's written even though you may have questions or even disagree with something. Follow it for six weeks, then make changes if you want.

Can I use condiments? Yes, including mayonnaise. Please do not buy any of the fat free mayonnaise either, unless you love the taste of it.

Fat free usually means high sugar.

Can I use salad dressings? Yes. The only salad dressings I do not like are those high in sugar, like flavored vinaigrettes. Same rule as above: Do not buy fat free dressings. One of my favorite snacks is to dip celery in blue cheese dressing.

What kind of cheese can I eat? Any kind you love!

Can I drink alcohol? My preference is that you eliminate alcohol for the first week or two while on the Extreme Burn Cycle to ensure you get off to a really fast start and get the results you're looking for. That said, I like to meet people where they are and create a win-win situation that allows you to fit this program into your life. If you decide not to give up alcohol, have it as part of your lunch meal on days 3, 5, 7, and count the calories as part of your 500-600 calories. I know what you're thinking, "I really like to enjoy a glass of wine or a beer in the evening to wind down, but not at lunch." I know the feeling, but I had to give this up to accomplish my goals. You can too.

Alcohol is metabolized very similarly to sugar, causing a rapid increase in blood sugars, which, in turn, elevates insulin levels. A common symptom of too much sugar or alcohol is increased abdominal fat. The great news is that you don't have to give it up forever!!! Once you have been on the program for a while, and your body has become an efficient fat burner, you can allow alcohol back in. Realize that to have the body you want, you may not be able to enjoy it quite as often, or in the quantities, you do now.

The best choice is red wine due to the high levels of resveratrol. I already explained in the chapter, Supplements, that resveratrol inhibits small fat cells from becoming large fat cells. I drink on occasion, and when I go out, I have vodka and a diet drink mix. Hard alcohol, by itself, does not contain that many calories; it's the mixer that add tons of sugar, so go diet.

Just as you can enjoy food and have the body you want, so can you enjoy alcohol. You just have to do it consciously. There may be periods of time you have to give it up altogether to get the body you want. The choice is up to you.

Do I have to use the supplements you recommend to see results? No. You can still see results on the Page Cycle without using supplements. I have recommended supplements long before I ever developed the Page Cycle. I feel strongly that no matter what program you're using to lose weight, for your general health, you will see better results using supplementation.

Where will I see results first? Typically, the first place you will see results is in your midsection. As I mentioned above, a side effect of high insulin levels is increased abdominal fat. A primary focus of the Page Cycle is to keep your blood sugars, and consequently your insulin levels, low.

Great news for the ladies! Before I developed the Page Cycle, the first place women normally would lose would be their breasts. I would get chewed out daily that, "now I have no breasts and my stomach looks even bigger." With the Page Cycle, your breasts will look even bigger as your waistline shrinks.

Nothing is more impactful on your health and your appearance than losing abdominal fat.

Can I exercise? Yes. More information will follow in the chapter on Exercise. The first week of the Extreme Burn Cycle, I recommend you do not exercise at all unless you are adamant that you need to. If you choose to exercise, decrease the intensity and duration by 50%. What you look like is 99% diet and 1% exercise. As always, the choice is yours.

How are beans classified? Beans are on my favorite foods and one of the best foods you can eat if you're looking to get lean. Beans have significant amounts of fiber and soluble fiber, with one cup of cooked beans providing between nine and 13 grams of fiber. Soluble fiber can help lower blood cholesterol. Beans are also high in protein, complex carbohydrates, folate, and iron.

With all of that said, for the purpose of the Page Cycle Diet beans are classified as a smart grain (carbohydrate). Beans have a-lot of protein but they also have a-lot of carbohydrates and should not be used on all protein days during The Extreme Burn Cycle.

Do all protein days mean zero carbs? All protein days do not mean zero carbs. Many of the foods you can eat on all protein days like cottage cheese, cheese, milk, peanut butter do contain what I call incidental carbohydrates. Take Skippy Natural Peanut Butter, the brand I use, for example: 2 TBSP has 6 grams of total carbohydrate two of which are fiber. The 6 grams of carbs are incidentals.

The goal is to keep the carbohydrates as low as possible not zero. On all protein days you can eat any of the foods in the protein & healthy fat lists even though they may contain "incidental" carbohydrates.

FIFTEEN

The Single Greatest Weight Management Tool: "Mini-Course Correction"

Pretty bold statement! In twenty years, I've literally used hundreds of techniques, tools, and strategies to assist people in losing body fat and keep it off.

A "mini course correction" is defined as one to two protein-only days. Sounds pretty simple, doesn't it? To be honest, the use of the "mini course correction" is the simplest and most effective weight management tool ever developed.

If I had a dollar for every person that told me, "I lost x number of pounds on x program, and kept it off until I went on a cruise (or vacation, or the holidays came, or I had a family reunion, or I had a two week period where I just got off track and couldn't get back on). Sound familiar?

Let's face it... These events are all a part of life. I love coaching new people on the Page Cycle. People call and text after only 24 to 48 hours, excited that they have lost weight. I'm always happy to hear that! But what I love as much as anything is when someone goes on vacation, gains five to ten pounds, and comes home and follows it up with a "mini-course correction." Then they tell me that they not only lost the weight they gained, but in most cases, lost additional weight as well. The freedom that person gains in that moment is truly life changing.

The pounds you gain from vacations, holidays, or a big cheat weekend are like relatives that come to stay with you. If you get rid of them quickly, there easy to get rid of, but if you let them hang around, you may never get rid of them.

Trust me when I tell you, the first time you experience how powerful the "mini-course correction" is, you will understand why I say, "it's the single greatest weight management tool ever developed."

Mini-Course Correction Protocol:

Use the first two days of the Extreme Burn Cycle after a binge week-end, vacation, or short period of overeating. It's recommended that if your eating has been off for more than one or two weeks, and you have gained a significant amount of weight, you should repeat a minimum of one Cycle of the Extreme Burn Cycle.

***Use mini course correction protocol as often as you would like to maintain your ideal weight....

"My husband and I just returned from vacation for a week. We were both in to the burn cycle already. Anyway, I was too freaked out to weigh when we got home but he did. He had gained 13 pounds as of Tuesday morning this week. We both went back on 2 days of protein and he is back down to exactly what he was before we went and I am down to within a pound. That is so cool!!!!! What a great testimony to the success of this way of life! Thank you so much for all your hard work and research that is life changing!" - Melissa Parker

SIXTEEN

Mike's 7 Laws of Leanness

Here are a few Laws, as I like to call them. If you follow these, they will guide you to a healthy lifestyle and allow you to maintain your weight once you reach your goal, as well as get you to your perfect size.

1. Start the day with at least of 10-30 grams of protein – When you're sleeping, your body starts to break down muscle tissue and use it as energy. When you wake up, your blood sugars are typically at their highest point in the day. Protein within thirty minutes of waking up stops the breakdown of muscle tissue and puts your body into a fat burning mode. Think of it as setting the tone for the day! You can either eat carbohydrates first thing and make your body an efficient fat storer, or start the day with protein and turn your body into a fat burning machine. The choice is yours!!!

2. Get at least half your body weight in grams of protein daily, spread out regularly, every three to four hours throughout the day. After approximately four hours without new protein your body will start to break down muscle tissue as energy. If you're

working out regularly, increase it to one gram per pound of body weight. Protein is critical in maintaining, or even increasing, your lean muscle tissue, which is your body's number one fat burning asset.

3. Get at least half your body weight in ounces of fluid daily. Adequate fluid intake improves digestion, increases metabolism, decreases hunger, aids in the elimination of toxins, and increases muscle tone. Dehydration can cause fatigue, headaches, and constipation, making weight loss difficult.

4. Limit or eliminate carbohydrates at night. Your body has the ability to eliminate excess fat and protein in your diet without increasing fat stores. The average person can store approximately 400-500 grams or 1600-2000 calories if your carbohydrate 'gas tank' is already full, and you eat carbohydrates at night, your body will store the excess carbohydrates as fat.

5. End the day with 10-30 grams of protein 30-60 minutes before bed. Traditional dieting wisdom says to eat at 6:00p.m. or 7:00p.m. and not to eat again. This is partially true; you don't want to eat carbohydrates at night, but you do want to eat protein. Protein before you go to sleep minimizes the breakdown of muscle tissue when you sleep.

6. Use "mini course corrections" to counteract binge eating, holidays, weekends, vacations, birthdays, or basically any time you eat excessive calories. Let's face it. Overeating is inevitable, but the weight gain is not. Those extra pounds are like house guests; if you only allow them to hang around for a day or two, they will come right off. If you let them stay awhile, they will be very difficult to get rid of.

7. Use the Page Cycle Diet, whether it's the Extreme Burn Cycle,

Burn Cycle, or the Steady Burn to stay lean for life. Routinely using food cycling will keep your metabolism elevated and allow you to enjoy food while looking the way you want.

SEVENTEEN

Do I Have To Exercise To Lose Weight On The Page Cycle?

I will tell you the same thing I've told every client who has sat down with me for the last twenty years. I can get you in the best shape of your life, but if you want to look differently, you're going to have to listen to me and change your nutrition.

What you look like is 99% nutrition and 1% exercise. I've literally had people spend $70,000 and look exactly the same as the day they started. They were in much better physical shape, felt better, and had dramatically improved their health, but at the end of the day, they did not really look much different. This really bothered me. In fact, ethically I struggled with this exact issue the last years of my personal training career.

I would provide people a free consultation, go over their goals, find out what their budget is, and lay out a plan for them. Nine times out of ten, people would choose to do the training, but would tell me they couldn't afford the nutritional supplements to get started on the fat burning program. I felt like saying, "I would rather see you spend your money on the supplements necessary to do the fat burning system, than spend your money on training."

I always felt like I was stuck between a rock and hard place. Ultimately, I decided to give up training for that exact reason. 99% of the clients that came to me wanted to look better through working out. I hope I have made it clear enough - how you look is based almost solely on your nutrition!

Just to give you an idea, it takes 3,500 calories to burn one pound of fat. Below is a short list of activities and how many calories each one burns. I did not include this to depress you; I did it to drive home the point that exercise has more to do with being in shape, and all the benefits that go along with that, than it does with losing weight. Based on this chart, it would take you 12.5 hours of windsurfing on the low end, and 2.2 hours of aggressive forestry ax chopping on the high end, to burn enough calories to burn a single pound of fat. On average a 150 lb person burns about 100 calories per mile running, which means they would burn about 2600 calories running a 26.2 mile marathon. Nine hundred calories short of burning 1 lb of fat.

I worked with hundreds of people who trained and completed a full 26.2 mile marathon. 95% of them gained body fat and lost muscle tissue by the time they completed their race. One of the hardest things for me to tell someone who loves to run is that if they want to look different, they're going to have to modify their training schedule.

I'm not saying you can't be a runner and look different. What I'm saying, if I have not made it clear enough, is that no matter how many calories you burn, you will not change your physical appearance if you are not eating to be lean. You cannot exercise away a bad diet!

The following chart can be found on at this URL: http://www.nutristrategy.com/activitylist4.htm

Exercise & Calories Burned per Hour

	130 lbs	155 lbs	180 lbs	205 lbs
Aerobics, general	384	457	531	605
Aerobics, high impact	413	493	572	651
Aerobics, low impact	295	352	409	465
Aerobics, step aerobics	502	598	695	791
Backpacking, Hiking with pack	413	493	572	651
Bagging grass, leaves	236	281	327	372
Ballet, twist, jazz, tap	266	317	368	419
Basketball, playing, non game	354	422	490	558
Bathing dog	207	246	286	326
Bowling	177	211	245	279
Boxing, punching bag	354	422	490	558
Calisthenics, light, push-ups, situps…	207	246	286	326
Calisthenics, fast, pushups, situps…	472	563	654	745
Canoeing, camping trip	236	281	327	372
Carrying small children	177	211	245	279
Children's games, hop-scotch…	295	352	409	465
Circuit training, minimal rest	472	563	654	745
Cleaning, dusting	148	176	204	233

Cross country skiing, moderate	472	563	654	745
Cycling, <10mph, leisure bicycling	236	281	327	372
Cycling, 10-11.9mph, light	354	422	490	558
Darts (wall or lawn)	148	176	204	233
Downhill snow skiing, moderate	354	422	490	558
Fishing, general	177	211	245	279
Football, touch, flag, general	472	563	654	745
Gardening, general	236	281	327	372
General cleaning	207	246	286	326
Golf, general	266	317	368	419
Gymnastics	236	281	327	372
Hacky sack	236	281	327	372
Handball	708	844	981	1117
Health club exercise	325	387	449	512
Hiking, cross country	354	422	490	558
Hockey, field hockey	472	563	654	745
Hockey, ice hockey	472	563	654	745
Horseback riding	236	281	327	372
Housework, light	148	176	204	233
Housework, moderate	207	246	286	326
Housework, vigorous	236	281	327	372
Hunting, general	295	352	409	465
Ice skating, average speed	413	493	572	651
Jai alai	708	844	981	1117
Jazzercise	354	422	490	558
Judo, karate, jujitsu, martial arts	590	704	817	931
Jumping rope, moderate	590	704	817	931

Kayaking	295	352	409	465
Kick boxing	590	704	817	931
Kickball	413	493	572	651
Krav maga class	590	704	817	931
Lacrosse	472	563	654	745
Masseur, masseuse, standing	236	281	327	372
Mild stretching	148	176	204	233
Mowing lawn, walk, power mower	325	387	449	512
Paddle boat	236	281	327	372
Paddleball, playing	354	422	490	558
Painting	266	317	368	419
Playing pool, billiards	148	176	204	233
Polo	472	563	654	745
Pushing stroller, walking with children	148	176	204	233
Race walking	384	457	531	605
Racquetball, playing	413	493	572	651
Raking lawn	254	303	351	400
Riding motorcyle	148	176	204	233
Rock climbing, ascending rock	649	774	899	1024
Rock climbing, mountain climbing	472	563	654	745
Rock climbing, rappelling	472	563	654	745
Roller blading, in-line skating	708	844	981	1117
Roller skating	413	493	572	651
Rowing machine, moderate	413	493	572	651
Rugby	590	704	817	931
Running, general	472	563	654	745

Sailing, yachting, ocean sailing	177	211	245	279
Shoveling snow by hand	354	422	490	558
Shuffleboard, lawn bowling	177	211	245	279
Skateboarding	295	352	409	465
Ski machine	413	493	572	651
Ski mobiling	413	493	572	651
Skiing, water skiing	354	422	490	558
Skindiving or scuba diving	708	844	981	1117
Sledding, tobagganing, luge	413	493	572	651
Snorkeling	295	352	409	465
Snow shoeing	472	563	654	745
Snow skiing, downhill skiing, light	295	352	409	465
Snowmobiling	207	246	286	326
Soccer, playing	413	493	572	651
Softball or baseball	295	352	409	465
Squash	708	844	981	1117
Stair machine	531	633	735	838
Stationary cycling, moderate	413	493	572	651
Stretching, hatha yoga	236	281	327	372
Surfing, body surfing or board surfing	177	211	245	279
Swimming, backstroke	413	493	572	651
Swimming, breaststroke	590	704	817	931
Swimming, butterfly	649	774	899	1024
Swimming laps, freestyle, fast	590	704	817	931
Swimming laps, freestyle, slow	413	493	572	651

Swimming leisurely, not laps	354	422	490	558
Swimming, sidestroke	472	563	654	745
Swimming, synchronized	472	563	654	745
Swimming, treading water, moderate	236	281	327	372
Table tennis, ping pong	236	281	327	372
Tae kwan do, martial arts	590	704	817	931
Tai chi	236	281	327	372
Taking out trash	177	211	245	279
Tennis playing	413	493	572	651
Track and field (high jump, pole vault)	354	422	490	558
Track and field (hurdles)	590	704	817	931
Track and field (shot, discus)	236	281	327	372
Trampoline	207	246	286	326
Volleyball, playing	177	211	245	279
Volleyball, beach	472	563	654	745
Walk / run, playing, moderate	236	281	327	372
Wallyball	413	493	572	651
Water aerobics	236	281	327	372
Weeding, cultivating garden	266	317	368	419
Weight lifting, body building, vigorous	354	422	490	558
Weight lifting, light workout	177	211	245	279
Whitewater rafting, kayaking,canoeing	295	352	409	465

| Windsurfing, sailing | 177 | 211 | 245 | 279 |
| Wrestling | 354 | 422 | 490 | 558 |

Even though nutrition and diet consist of 99% of the change you can make for your body, exercise can also aid in your weight loss journey, and the additional benefits from exercise are numerous.

Exercise Benefit #1: Increased energy. The right combination of exercise and nutrition creates a hormonal environment conducive to fat loss, increased muscle strength, and increased energy. When your body is working at peak efficiency, your energy levels soar! Everyday things become much easier to do.

Exercise Benefit #2: Increased Self-Esteem. Gaining control of your body size and weight through fitness is an amazing way to increase self-esteem. You look better and are more confident, which empowers you in everything you do. You will find that the self-discipline required and learned through regular exercise spills over into other areas of your life, and you will be better able to make other necessary and desirable changes.

Exercise Benefit #3: Increased Mental Focus. Did you know that the latest research shows that exercise helps keep your brain sharp, well into old age? Anything that involves mental acuity (focus and concentration) is improved. You also stand a much better chance of avoiding such diseases as Alzheimer's and senility.

Exercise Benefit #4: Decreased Risk of a Heart Attack. By exercising regularly and making positive changes in your diet, you lower your cholesterol and blood pressure and greatly diminish the chances of having a heart attack.

Exercise Benefit #5: Decreased Risk of Osteoporosis. Regular exercise, especially weight-bearing exercise, reduces the risk of osteoporosis, and can even reverse it by building bone tissue!

Exercise Benefit #6: Reduced Risk of Breast Cancer by up to 60%. Estradiol and progesterone, two ovarian hormones linked to breast cancer tumor production, are lowered in the body by exercise.

A woman's body is most susceptible to these hormones during the time between ovulation and menstruation. Habitual exercise can actually delay ovulation until later in the menstrual cycle. This reduces the time she must fight these hormones.

Fat has long been known to be a catalyst in the production of estrogen (estradiol). Regular exercise burns body fat and, thus, decreases the rate of estrogen production.

So there you have it! A two pronged, cancer preventing, exercise benefit!

Exercise Benefit #7: Increased Strength and Stamina. Every physical thing you do becomes easier, which is immensely useful in everyday life.

Exercise Benefit #8: Reduced Depression. The production of endorphins ("feel good" hormones) is increased through exercise. Nothing improves mood and suppresses depression better than those endorphins.

Exercise Benefit #9: Decreased Stress Levels. The worries and stresses of everyday living (commuting, work demands, conflicts, etc.) can stick with you long after the workday is done. Exercising right after work is the perfect natural therapy that can change your mood. You will sleep better, too!

Exercise Benefit #10: Well, actually, here are another fifty benefits...

- Improved digestion.
- Enhanced quality of sleep.
- Added sparkle and radiance to complexion.
- Improved body shape.
- Helps with toned and firm muscles.
- More muscular definition.

- Enables weight loss and keeps it off, which makes it easier to qualify for affordable health insurance.
- Makes you limber.
- Improves endurance.
- Burns extra calories.
- Improves circulation and helps reduce blood pressure.
- Increases lean muscle tissue in the body.
- Improves appetite for healthy foods.
- Alleviates menstrual cramps.
- Alters and improves muscle chemistry.
- Increases metabolic rate.
- Enhances coordination and balance.
- Improves posture.
- Eases, and possibly eliminates, back problems and pain.
- Makes the body use calories more efficiently.
- Lowers resting heart rate.
- Increases muscle size through an increase in muscle fibers.
- Improves body composition.
- Increases body density.
- Decreases fat tissue more easily.
- Makes body more agile.
- Is the greatest body tune-up.
- Reduces joint discomfort.
- Improves athletic performance.
- Enriches sexuality.
- May add a few years to life.
- Increases your range of motion.
- Enhances immune system.
- Improves glycogen storage.

- Enables the body to utilize energy more efficiently.
- Increases enzymes in the body that burn fat.
- Increases the number and size of mitochondria in muscle cells.
- Increases concentration of myoglobin (carries oxygen in muscles) in skeletal muscles.
- Enhances oxygen transport throughout the body.
- Improves liver functioning.
- Increases speed of muscle contraction and reaction time.
- Enhances feedback through the nervous system.
- Strengthens the heart.
- Improves blood flow.
- Helps to alleviate varicose veins.
- Increases maximum cardiac output.
- Increases contractility of the heart's ventricles.
- Increases the weight and size of the heart.
- Improves contractile function of the whole heart.
- Makes calcium transport in the heart and body more efficient.

Now that we are clear that exercise has a million and one benefits, and that it will aid in your weight loss journey, let me give you a quick down-and-dirty guide to optimize your results.

As your personal weight loss coach, I encourage you to make exercise part of your overall weight loss plan for life. If you choose to make exercise part of your life, I want to make sure you are maximizing your results and spending time on the activities that produce results.

Weight training is king. The key to having a lean, sexy body is muscle tissue. When you weight train, you break down muscle tissue, causing an increase in metabolism. As you continue to break down muscle tissue, the body's response is to build more muscle tissue. The more muscle tissue you have, the faster your metabolism will be, resulting in greater fat loss.

The effect of weight training is a faster metabolism 24 hours a day, 365 days a year. I spend 99% of the time at the gym doing weight training because it's the key to my goals. No hours of boring cardio for me.

One pound of muscle tissue burns between 35 and 50 calories per day. An increase of five pounds of muscle tissue leads to significant increases in calories burned. 5 x 50 x 365 = 91,250 more calories burned per year! In theory, this equals 26 pounds of fat loss per year.

Over the past twenty years, approximately 80% of my clients have been women who, before they met me, had never really lifted weights. The most common question I would get asked was, "will lifting weights make me bulky?" The answer is no! For 99.999% of the population, and especially women, lifting weights will not make you bulky. In fact, lifting weights will do the exact opposite: it will give you a smaller, more petite body.

More and more research is advocating weight training as the key to fat loss. Fitness Management Magazine conducted a study to determine the role of weight training on body composition changes. In this study, 72 overweight men and women were divided into two groups. Both ate the same diets and exercised 30 minutes a day for eight weeks. One group followed a typical weight-loss exercise program, spending all thirty minutes on aerobic exercise, while the second group did fifteen minutes of aerobic exercise (exercycling) and fifteen minutes of weight training (Nautilus machines). Here are the results:

Exercise Program	Body Weight Changes	Fat Weight Changes	Muscle Weight Changes
Endurance exercise only	-3.5 pounds	-3.0 pounds	-0.5 pounds
Endurance and strength exercise	-8.0 pounds	-10.0 pounds	+2.0 pounds

As you can see, the group that performed strength training lost over three times as much body fat as the group that only performed aerobic exercise. There is absolutely no doubt whether or not exercise, and especially strength training, is beneficial in losing body fat and weight.

Even with these numbers, know that you don't have to exercise in order to see results. Will you see even better results if you add exercise to your overall program? Yes. Do I hope you choose to incorporate exercise into your program? Yes. Do you have to exercise to see results on the Page Cycle? Absolutely not. In fact, I spend as much time counseling people to not exercise as much as I do counseling people to get started on an exercise program.

Aerobic exercise: In my experience, 99% of the population believes that aerobic exercise is the key to losing weight. The infomercial world has done an amazing job creating a belief that if you can burn enough calories, you will lose weight and have that lean sexy body.

From the chart above, you can see that a 205lb. person doing general running burns approximately 800 calories per hour. Mathematically, this equates to approximately 4.5 hours of running to burn one pound of fat.

One of the most common questions I get asked about aerobic training is, "If I want to burn fat, what is the best intensity to do my cardio at?" That is not a simple question. I'm going to give you the long version so that you fully understand this subject.

When our bodies are at rest, we are burning primarily fat. To simplify matters, let's say that, at rest, our bodies are burning 100% fat. The moment we start to exercise, the percentage of fat we are burning starts to decrease.

The percentage of fat we burn decreases proportionately the harder we exercise,. Get on any treadmill in any gym and almost all of them will have a graph that shows your heart rate in comparison to the percentage of fat being burned. The graph will show a corresponding range for your heart rate that is optimal to burn fat.

Marketers have done a fantastic job at selling this story and, in reality, they are telling the truth. However, when we take a look at the other side of the story, they are misleading people to believe the best way to burn fat is to exercise moderately.

The other side of the story is that the harder you exercise, the more calories you burn. I love examples, so let's take a look at Bill, a runner, and see in which workout Bill burns more fat.

Bill - Weight: 205	
Running @ 5 mph	Running @ 10 mph
Calories Burned/hr – 745 cal	Calories burned/hr – 1489 cal
% of fat burned 60% - 447 cal	% of fat burned 40% - 595 cal

In the above example, not only did Bill burn almost twice as many calories overall, but he also burned 25% more fat calories.

The biggest mistake I see people making in the gym is that they're not working hard enough. If you can manage to read a book while walking on the treadmill, it is a good clue you're not working hard enough.

Your body will adapt to the stress that you place upon it. If you exercise at a lower intensity to burn more fat, your body responds by storing more fat so that it can meet the demands of what you're asking it to do.

The key to aerobic exercise is short duration, high intensity workouts. The stress you're placing on your body signals it to give up fat stores and store more muscle glycogen to meet the demands you're placing upon it.

This is the exact opposite of what most people believe because of the message that clever marketers use to sell their current gadget or gizmo. Take a look at sprinters, for example. The longest duration they ever maintain is approximately ninety seconds at a time; they have some of the most beautiful lean bodies in the world.

My personal preference is to do interval training. Interval training allows you to do periods of high intensity, combined with low intensity. I have used and recommended interval training almost exclusively for 20 years.

Here is a sample workout plan I like to do. The ratings are based on a rating of perceived exertion with 1 being the easiest and ten being the hardest. The intensity is high and the workout is short and sweet!!!

2 min. level 5, 1 min. level 6, 1 min. level 7, 1 min. level 8, 1 min. level 5, 1 min. level 6, 1 min. level 7, 1 min. level 8, 1 min. level 5, 1 min. level 6, 1 min. level 7, 1 min. level 8, 1 min. level 5, 1 min. level 6, 1 min. level 7, 1 min. level 8, 1 min. level 9, 2 min. level 5, 20 min. total.

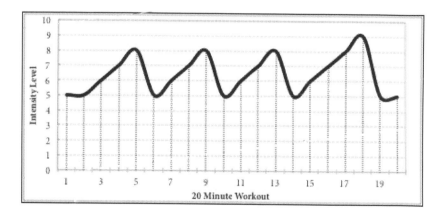

***One thing I want to make sure you understand is that I'm not saying you should never do long, slow aerobics, or utilize different intensities. I believe you should constantly switch things up. What I'm saying is that the majority of time spent doing aerobics should be at a high intensity.

Modifying Workouts While On The Page Cycle

If you're currently exercising, or decide to begin an exercise program in conjunction with the Page Cycle Diet, I have a couple of recommendations and modifications for you.

Decrease your exercise intensity and duration by 50% during your first seven days on Extreme Burn. On Extreme Burn, you're depleting all of the carbohydrates (glycogen) which are the primary fuel source used during exercise. If you work out as hard as you usually do before your body has adapted to burning primarily fat, it won't turn out so well. It's very common for people to get dizzy and nauseated if they do not reduce the intensity. I usually tell people to take the first week off or, if they feel they cannot stop, to at least reduce the intensity and duration.

Once you have gone through the first seven day Extreme Burn Cycle, you can resume your full intensity workouts without any problems. Your body will be much more efficient at burning fat as a fuel source. Many people find they are able to exercise at a much higher intensity within a short period of time.

***As your body becomes more efficient at burning fat (an almost unlimited supply of energy) as a fuel source during exercise, instead of glycogen (a very limited supply), you will find that you can work out harder and longer.

EIGHTEEN

Plateau Busters And Maintenance Strategies

These strategies have been used with thousands of people over the last twenty years to break through plateaus and continue to have success. One thing to realize about these strategies is that you can use them in a way that fits into your life and maximizes your results. The whole point of the Page Cycle, and these strategies, is to make them fit your lifestyle and allow you to enjoy food and still get the results you want. Everyone's body responds differently, and in the end, each person has to create strategies that work for them.

Two Day Binge

The Page Cycle is so amazing at controlling hunger that sometimes, on the quest to lose weight and get leaner, it's easy to decrease calories to a point where the body goes into a protection mode. When in protection mode, the body will slow down the metabolism and conserve fat stores, no matter how few calories you eat.

Protocol: The two day binge is exactly what it sounds like. Eat like you will never eat again!!! Do not worry if the foods are healthy or not, just eat! This strategy is best used if you find yourself never hungry; generally, this means your metabolism has slowed down too much. Two days of eating excess calories will be enough to make your body feel comfortable again, and allow you to continue to lose weight and body fat. It's best if followed by at least one week of the Extreme Burn Cycle.

Protein Only After 3:00P.M.

Extremely powerful strategy to utilize if you have hit a plateau!!!

Protocol: Do not eat carbohydrates after 3:00p.m. There are two primary ways to utilize this strategy. First, use it to break through plateaus by adopting it for 7-21 days. Second, utilize this strategy as a maintenance tool by adopting this strategy 4-5 days a week, allowing you to maintain your weight and have more freedom throughout the day.

Junk Food Special

Everyone has those times where nothing will do but their favorite high calorie special treat. Whether it is a bloomin' onion (over 3,000 calories) from Outback Steakhouse or a hamburger, fries, and a large soda from your favorite fast food joint (about 2,000 calories), sometimes you just have to give in to get it out of your system. If you do it right, you can use it to spur your weight loss to new heights.

Protocol: Do not use for longer than four or five days! Start off the day with a pure protein source. By two o'clock, have your favorite junk food meal and cut your eating off at that time. You will be able to have your favorite meal and still stay within your calorie range if you do not eat anything the rest of the day and evening. You can have a protein-only meal in the evening on these days to satisfy any hunger you may feel. This strategy allows you to feed your cravings and not go overboard. After a few days, you will most likely be tired of eating whatever high fat, high calorie food you have been eating. Sometimes our bodies and minds just need to be satisfied. Follow up this strategy by repeating the Extreme Burn Cycle one to two times for maximum results.

Go Offline

Sometimes it's a good idea to eat what you want, when you want, and to not pay attention to the scale for a week or two. The body can get used to whatever you're doing, and to break that cycle, discontinue all your weight loss efforts to give yourself a break mentally and physically.

Protocol: Discontinue the Page Cycle for one to two weeks. Follow it up with one to two cycles of The Extreme Burn Cycle.

Burn, Baby

Start an exercise program if you are not currently exercising.

Protocol: Start an exercise program with a goal in mind to burn 500 calories a day, three to six days a week. Choose aerobic activities like walking, running, biking, etc., that get the heart rate up and maximize the number of calories burned for the time spent. Add weight training to raise your resting metabolism, which lets you burn more calories 24 hours a day, 365 days a year.

Food Journal

If you hit a plateau, one of the best ways to figure out what is going on is to write down everything you eat for a couple weeks. You may find that even though you think you have been doing a great job choosing low calorie, healthy options, one or two bad habits are killing your weight loss success.

Protocol: Go online and search the keywords, free online diet journal. You will find a bunch of choices. Play with a couple and set up an online journal that you can keep for a few weeks. The biggest key is that it will educate you on the caloric value of food so that you can make smart choices in any situation.

***The strategies listed above are tools that you can use to create a lifestyle that works for you.

***Realize that weight loss is not always a straight line process, and that if you are in a plateau, it is not necessarily a bad thing. Shake things up and use one or more of the strategies above to stimulate your body to reach a new level of weight loss.

Simple Strategies To Keep The Weight Off

Set a five pound weight-gain mark – You worked your tail off to get to your ideal weight, so work as hard to keep it there. Once you hit the five pound weight-gain mark, go back on The Extreme Burn Cycle immediately, no matter what occasions may be coming up. One thing is for sure, holidays, birthdays, and other events will always be there to try and make you stumble. Just make a decision not to let it happen.

Continue using the products on a regular basis – Use the products every day to maintain your ideal weight. I am a firm believer in continuing to do the activities that created success in the first place. I use supplements every day and believe they are a big part of my success.

Mini Course Corrections – The reality of life is that we all have times when we eat more than we should: holidays, birthdays, vacation, etc… Whatever the reasons are, everyone falls off the wagon from time to time. The use of a "mini course correction" is the perfect way to get back on track fast, re-ignite your metabolism, and get rid of extra pounds in short order.

See Chapter on "Mini Course Corrects."

Protein-only dinners: three or four nights a week, make it a habit to have protein-only dinners. The Page Cycle teaches that excess carbs, especially at night, will lead to unwanted fat storage.

Eat six small meals per day: Get in the habit of eating more frequent meals and to include a small amount of protein in each one. Eating small, more frequent meals stimulates the body's metabolism and makes it easier to maintain ideal weight.

Create an online food journal: This is a very valuable tool if you have had trouble maintaining your weight in the past. It is very easy to get in the habit of eating too many calories daily. Take the time to create an online food journal which will not only tell you how many calories you are eating daily, but gives you an incredible education in the caloric value of the foods you frequently eat.

Read food labels: Get in the habit of reading every food label you can get your hands on. Education is a big key in maintaining your ideal weight. Many of the foods "coined" as healthy are really nothing more than high calorie foods that will make it difficult to maintain your ideal weight. Fruit juice is a prime example of a food thought of as healthy that is actually packed with sugar and calories.

Do an Extreme Burn Cycle every sixty days: We all probably get regular oil changes and maintenance on our vehicle. Our bodies are no different! You may be at your ideal weight and feel like everything is going great, but if you want to make sure your body is firing on all cylinders, do an Extreme Burn Cycle every sixty days.

Create a weekly schedule: A weekly schedule has to work for your life, but must also keep you on track with your weight loss goals, whether it's losing or maintaining your weight. This schedule has to be one that you can work with for a lifetime! The whole point of the schedule is to be able to have days built in when you can eat whatever you want, in whatever quantities you want, followed by protein-only days to keep you at your ideal weight.

NINETEEN

~~~~~~

Ten Fat Burning Meals

~~~~~~

People are always asking me what to eat? I have ten meals that are ideal for losing weight; they can be used on meal days, and several can be used for protein-only days as well. I added these recipes to give you some ideas. Take any of the items on your food list provided, and create whatever meals you enjoy (for each appropriate day).

I have always told my clients that eating healthy and eating to be lean are two different things. For example, the next time you go to the store, pick up a box of granola cereal and compare the nutritional information to a box of Kashi. This is just one example of how one choice in your day, between two healthy items, can make the difference between eating to be lean or not.

Take twenty minutes and go to the internet and search high protein, low calorie meals, cereals, snacks, etc… Find foods that you enjoy eating. Replace the foods in your diet that are high calorie, low nutrient with foods you love that arc low calorie, high nutrition.

You should never get bored! The possibilities are endless, only limited by your imagination. Most of the time, I keep my meals pretty simple. For me, the key to variety is using all sorts of pre-made sauces and lots of spices.

One last note: On protein-only days, utilize healthy fats (nuts, avocados, healthy oils, seeds, peanut butter, almond butter, mayonnaise, low sugar salad dressings, [i.e. blue cheese, ranch, thousand island] to add flavor, enjoyment, and nutritional value. The Page Cycle is not a low fat, deprivation diet. Enjoy the foods you're eating!!!

Quick 'N Easy Balsamic Chicken
(Protein-only day or meal day)
High Protein, Low Fat Heart-Healthy Food Option
25 Minutes to Prepare and Cook

Ingredients

1 Chicken Breast (cut in thin 2-inch strips)

4 Tbsp Balsamic Vinegar

2 tsp freshly chopped garlic

1 tsp Olive Oil

Salt and Pepper to taste

Directions

1. Cut chicken breast in thin 2-inch strips
2. Chop fresh garlic - about 2 tsp (about 4-5 cloves of garlic)
3. Heat oil in a pan and add garlic. Saute until golden.
4. Add chicken and stir well.
5. Add Balsamic vinegar and salt and pepper.
6. Reduce the heat to medium and let the excess water evaporate.
7. Keep stirring intermittently, making sure that all the water dries

up and the chicken is well coated with Balsamic Vinegar.

8.   Serve hot with some brown rice or whole wheat pasta.

Nutritional Info:

Calories: 166.5

Total Fat: 5.4 g

Cholesterol: 41.2 mg

Sodium: 222.2 mg

Total Carbs: 9.9 g

Dietary Fiber: 0.1 g

Protein: 16.8 g Protein

Easy Turkey Chili

Done in less than 30 minutes and super healthy

45 Minutes to Prepare and Cook

Ingredients

1 pound lean ground turkey (93% lean)

2C chopped onion

1C chopped celery

1C chopped bell pepper

6 cloves chopped garlic

2T olive oil

1 can black beans

2 can kidney beans

1 can pinto beans

2 cans diced tomatoes

1 quart chicken broth

Chili powder to taste

Directions

I split this up into eight 2-cup servings, and it still is low in calories and fat, and high in protein!

Brown ground turkey in 1T olive oil, sauté onion, celery, bell pepper and garlic in 1T olive oil. Add remaining ingredients and simmer for 15 minutes or longer to taste. Add chili powder, salt, and pepper to taste.

Number of Servings: 8

Nutritional Info:

Calories: 312.3

Total Fat: 9.3 g

Cholesterol: 41.3 mg

Sodium: 1,240.3 mg

Total Carbs: 33.3 g

Dietary Fiber: 10.7 g

Protein: 25.4 g

Protein Pancakes

High Protein, Low Carb Pancakes.

20 Minutes to Prepare and Cook

Ingredients

1 Whole Egg (*2 egg whites or 1/4 C. Egg Beaters)

1/4 C. Fat Free Cottage Cheese

1/4 C. Old Fashioned Oatmeal (powdered in blender if preferred)

1 Scoop of vanilla, chocolate, plain protein powder

Vanilla or Maple Extract to Taste

Ground Cinnamon to Taste

Water

Directions

Blend all ingredients together in a blender until it forms a batter-like consistency.

Spray a non-stick skillet with cooking spray & cook batter into 3 pancakes.

Optional: Peanut butter and Splenda are my toppings of choice.

These taste great!! I usually make 4+ recipes & cook them all. Then I freeze them & pop in the microwave for a quick breakfast.

Number of Servings: 3

Nutritional Info:

Calories: 73.9

Total Fat: 2.4 g

Cholesterol: 71.7 mg

Sodium: 54.9 mg

Total Carbs: 5.1 g

Dietary Fiber: 0.8 g

Protein: 7.8 g

Salmon Salad

High in protein, low in carbs and calories!

5 Minutes to Prepare and Cook

Ingredients

2 cups salmon, flaked

1 red or yellow bell pepper, diced

1 cucumber, peeled, seeded & diced

.5 cup chopped onion

4-5 tbsp. greek yogurt, plain (enough to moisten)

1/4 tsp. cayenne pepper

Salt & pepper

Juice of 1/2 a lemon

*Optional: 2 hardboiled eggs (not included in nutritional information)

Directions

In a large bowl, gently toss together the salmon and crushed hard-boiled eggs (optional). In another bowl, combine bell pepper, cucumber, onion, and yogurt. Add seasonings and stir to combine. Pour mixture over salmon, add lemon juice, and toss lightly to combine. Serve over lettuce or as a sandwich.

Number of Servings: 4

Nutritional Info

Calories: 188.4

Total Fat: 6.2 g

Cholesterol: 20.0 mg

Sodium: 347.9 mg

Total Carbs: 4.9 g

Dietary Fiber: 1.0 g

Protein: 26.1 g

Turkey Soufflé

(Protein or meal day) Ideal Protein day if you take the flour out.
Filling low-carb, high-protein meal!

Ingredients

2 cups fresh turkey breast meat - cubed

9 medium eggs, whites/yolks separated

9 tbsp white flour (whole wheat flour can be substituted)

9 tbsp margarine

1 tsp black pepper

1 tsp salt

Directions

Melt margarine in at least a 2 qt saucepan and slowly add flour, stirring constantly until mixture is creamy.

Turn off stove.

Slowly add egg yolks and whites continue stirring as the mixture cools slightly.

Stir in cubed turkey breast meat until thoroughly mixed. Pour mixture into a greased 4-6 qt. baking dish.

Bake uncovered at 350° for 45 minutes, or until the top is slightly browned and/or a knife comes out clean from the center of the soufflé.

**Recipe can be divided into thirds for smaller serving needs.

Number of Servings: 12

Nutritional Info:

Calories: 159.9   Total Carbs: 7.4 g

Total Fat: 9.7 g   Dietary Fiber: 0.4 g

Cholesterol: 149.4 mg   Protein: 8.6 g

Sodium: 518.7 mg

Tuna Patty Melt

(Protein day or meal day)

Low fat/calorie, high protein alternative to a beef or chicken burger.

15 Minutes to Prepare and Cook

Ingredients

1 Can of Tuna (drained)

1 Egg White

1/3 Cup of Low Fat Cheddar Cheese

1/2 Small Onion (Finely Chopped)

1 tsp Ground Garlic

1/2 tsp Pepper

Directions

In a bowl mix drained tuna, egg white, cheese, onion and spices until all the ingredients stick together.

Split in half and form two patties.

In a medium saucepan, fry patties until both sides are golden brown.

Number of Servings: 2

Nutritional Info:

Calories: 98.0

Total Fat: 1.9 g

Cholesterol: 28.9 mg

Sodium: 392.5 mg

Total Carbs: 2.1 g

Dietary Fiber: 0.3 g

Protein: 18.3 g

Cream of Broccoli and Cauliflower Soup

Protein Packed

40 Minutes to Prepare and Cook

Just one serving of this creamy soup contains 1 serving of vegetables, 1 serving of milk, 4 grams of fiber, 17 grams of protein, and more than a day's supply of Vitamin C.

Ingredients

1 lb mixture of broccoli and cauliflower (or substitute broccoli or broc-

coflower) coarsely chopped (about 2 cups)

6 scallions (green onions), chopped

2 cups Vegetable Broth

1 garlic clove, minced

1 cup nonfat evaporated milk

40 grams vegetable protein powder (optional**)

2 Tbs Smart Balance 37% Light Buttery Spread

1 tsp dried Marjoram

1 tsp black pepper

Directions

- Combine broth, broccoli/cauliflower mixture (save about 1/3 cup of broccoli for later!), garlic, and scallions in a saucepan. Bring to a boil. Reduce heat and simmer covered for about 10 minutes until veggies are tender.
- Remove from heat and cool for a few minutes. Transfer to a blender or food processor and puree until smooth.
- Steam the remaining 1/3 cup of broccoli in the microwave. Finely chop.
- In the saucepan, melt the margarine. Mix in marjoram and pepper. Gradually stir in milk until smooth. Cook over medium heat, stirring, until thick and bubbling.
- Add the pureed soup and broccoli to milk mixture and heat to serving temperature.
- Salt and pepper to taste.

Makes 4 servings

Nutritional Info

Calories: 149.5

Total Fat: 3.0 g

Cholesterol: 2.6 mg

Sodium: 416.8 mg

Total Carbs: 15.3 g

Dietary Fiber: 4.0 g

Protein: 16.8 g

On The Go Breakfast Cookies

Quick high protein high fiber breakfast/snack

17 Minutes to Prepare and Cook

Ingredients

16 tbsp. Flax Seed Meal (ground flax)

8 tsp. Splenda Brown Sugar Blend

1 cup Peanut Butter, chunk style

1 tsp Baking Soda

2 large Eggs, fresh

Directions

Preheat oven to 350 . Mix flax and baking soda together, then add egg mix with peanut butter unti creamy. Teaspoon onto and bake on a no-stick baking pan for 12 minutes.

2 cookies per serving.

Number of Servings: 12

Nutritional Info

Calories: 192.3

Total Fat: 14.6 g

Cholesterol: 35.4 mg

Sodium: 219.8 mg

Total Carbs: 10.1 g

Dietary Fiber: 4.4 g

Protein: 8.2 g

Low Carb Egg And Cottage Cheese Salad

Protein day leave out salad / Meal day with salad

An easy low fat and low carb egg salad with no mayo at all!

35 Minutes to Prepare and Cook

Ingredients

2 hard boiled eggs (one yolk can be removed)

1/3 cup 1% cottage cheese

Salt (seasoned salt is best flavor with egg)

Pepper

(Add a little dill, dijon mustard or other favorite to give this a little more flavor.)

Directions

Hard boil eggs and remove one of the yolks to lower the fat. Chop egg whites and one yolk. Mix in cottage cheese, and season to taste. You will have a high protein low fat egg salad in no time.

Number of Servings: 1

Nutritional Info

Calories: 148.2

Total Fat: 6.2 g

Cholesterol: 215.0 mg

Sodium: 419.8 mg

Total Carbs: 2.8 g

Dietary Fiber: 0.0 g

Protein: 20.5 g

Low Carb, High Protein Taco Bake

(Protein or meal day)

You can serve with additional toppings like shredded lettuce, jalapenos, guacamole, ripe olives, sour cream or salsa, but be sure to add in your nutrition info.

Ingredients

Crust

> 4 ounces fat free cream cheese, softened
>
> 3 egg whites
>
> 1/3 cup Fat free half and half
>
> 1/2 teaspoon taco seasoning
>
> 8 ounces low fat cheddar cheese, shredded

Topping

> 1 lb ground turkey, 93% lean
>
> 3 teaspoons taco seasoning
>
> 1/4 cup tomato sauce
>
> 4 ounces chopped green chilies
>
> 8 ounces cheddar cheese, shredded

Directions

- For the crust, beat the cream cheese and eggs until smooth.
- Add the cream and seasoning.
- Grease a 9"x13" baking dish; spread the cheese over the bottom.
- Pour in the egg mixture as evenly as possible.
- Bake at 375ºF, 25-30 minutes.
- Let stand 5 minutes before adding the topping.
- For the topping, brown the hamburger; drain fat.

- Stir in the seasoning, tomato sauce and chiles.
- Spread over the crust.
- Top with cheese.
- Reduce oven to 350ºF and bake another 20 minutes or so until hot and bubbly.
- Serve with the toppings of your choice (add additional carbs).

Makes 8 servings.

Nutritional Info

Calories: 160.8	Total Carbs: 3.7 g
Total Fat: 6.4 g	Dietary Fiber: 0.2 g
Cholesterol: 47.5 mg	Protein: 22.2 g
Sodium: 449.3 mg	

TWENTY

10 Fat Burning Snacks

Here are ten snacks that will help you get started and get you through your day.

Beef jerky

Believe it or not, this old classic is actually a healthy choice. On average, one ounce contains about 70 calories and one gram of fat, but delivers 11 grams of protein. If you have concerns about high sodium, you can look for low sodium versions in health food stores.

Eggs

For only 70 calories each, eggs are rich in nutrients. They contain, in varying amounts, almost every essential vitamin and mineral needed by humans, as well as several other beneficial food components. A large egg contains over six grams of protein. A large egg has 4.5 grams of fat, only 7% of the daily value. Only one-third (1.5 grams) is saturated fat, and 2 grams are mono-, unsaturated fat!

Cottage cheese and fruit

A half cup of 2% cottage cheese contains, on average, 16 grams of protein, yet only has 102 calories and two grams of fat. Add veggies or fruit on higher carbohydrate days or enjoy as a standalone on protein-only days.

Tuna

Tuna is a great source of protein, with approximately 25 grams per can. Plus, one can of tuna in water contains approximately 111 calories and is fat-free.

Nuts

Nuts, which still high in fat, are AWESOME sources of protein and are very easy to throw in an airtight container.

Deli Meat

Make sure you choose whole cuts that do not contain nitrates and are unprocessed. Nothing is easier than throwing a serving of your favorite deli meat in a baggy or tupperware to eat on the go.

Lentils

Although they may not seem appetizing on their own, putting a handful of them in your soup or salad will give your snack a protein boost. One cup of lentils has about 230 calories, one gram of fat, and 18 grams of protein.

Peanut butter

If you loved peanut butter and jelly sandwiches as a kid, you're in luck: one tablespoon contains about four grams of protein, eight grams of fat, and 95 calories. For an energy boost, spread it on a slice of whole-wheat bread (60 calories and one gram of fat), and top it with banana slices.

CARBmaster Yogurt (Kroger brand)

I love the taste, and with only 80 calories, 4 grams of carbohydrates, and a whopping 12 grams of protein, this is an ideal fat-burning snack.

Edamame

Dry roasted edamame is something you can pack in your purse or gym bag. Each ¼ cup only has 140 calories, but a whopping 14 grams of protein, making it a low calorie fat burning snack.

163

TWENTY-ONE

Final Thoughts

I know that you're probably really excited to get started. I also know you may have some fears, concerns, and questions. I've been in your shoes before. It's okay to feel what you're feeling, but it's not okay to allow these emotions and feelings to keep you from having the life you want. Actively create more pain in being heavier than you would like than in the fear and/or limiting thoughts that have held you back in the past. Make a commitment to follow the Page Cycle Diet 100% for twelve weeks, and I promise your life will never be the same.

I want you to know that I'm in this with you. Nothing would make me happier than to hear about your success, so e-mail me at success@pagecyclediet.com. When I developed the Page Cycle Diet four years ago, my goal was to empower ten million people to lose 100 million pounds. I had no idea how I was going to achieve my goal until I met a man who shared my same vision. I believe the only way for people to have success and keep the weight off long term is to learn the truth about losing weight (body fat).

I will continue to provide education and support to anyone who is following my plan. Please visit my website www.pagecyclediet.com often as I will continue to improve the support I provide or to get more information on supplements I recommend.

I know the Page Cycle Diet works. Not just for some people, but for everybody. The only variable in this equation is you. I believe in you and I know that you can reach your goal.

Appendix

The Glycemic Index

Glycemic Index, or GI Index, is a ranking of carbohydrates on a scale from 0 to 100 according to the extent to which they raise blood sugar levels. It measures how much your blood glucose increases after eating a meal.

Low Glycemic Index foods (less than 55) produce a small rise in blood sugar and insulin level. Foods with GI index between 55 and 70 are consider intermediate-GI foods. High Glycemic Index food GI numbers (more than 70) make our blood sugar and insulin levels rise fast.

One of the keys to keeping your body in a fat burning mode is to keep the insulin levels in your body low. The key to doing that is to choose foods that are low on the glycemic index. As you can see, vegetables and protein are the best choices.

Category	Food Name	Glycemic Index
Vegetables		
	Baked Beans, 4oz.	48
	Kidney beans, 3 oz.	27
	Lima beans, 3 oz.	32
	Navy beans, 3 oz.	38
	Pinto beans, 4oz.	45
	Soy beans, 3 oz.	18
	Beets, 3 oz.	64

Category	Food Name	Glycemic Index
	Tomato Sauce	49
	Peas	48
	Sweetcorn	48
	Broccoli, cauliflower, celery	10-25
	Vegetarian chili	39
	Mashed potato, instant	74
	French Fries, baked	54
	Potato, peeled & steamed	65
	Carrots	47
Breads		
	Dark rye, 1.7 oz.	51
	French baguette, 1 oz.	95
	Hamburger bun, 1 bun	61
	Kaiser roll, 1	73
	Pita bread – whole wheat, 1 slice	57
	Sourdough, 1 slice	52
	Fruit Bread	53
	White bread, 1 slice	70
	Wonder Bread, White Enriched	71
	Wheat bread – stoneground, 1 slice	53
	Whole wheat, 1 slice	69
	Bagel, plain, white, 2 oz.	72
	Wholegrain Bread	40
	Multigrain Breads	45
	English Muffin, Whole Grain	45
	Oat Bread	65
	Rye Bread	50
	Bran Muffin	65
Meats / Chicken		
	Sweet & Sour Chicken w/Noodles	41
	Lean Cuisine, French style Chicken	36
	Beef casserole	53

Category	Food Name	Glycemic Index
	Chicken Nuggets, frozen	46
	Fish Fingers (strips)	38
	Pizza, cheese	60
	Sausages	28
	Hamburger (with bun)	66
	Chicken Nuggets, frozen & microwaved	46
	Sushi, roasted	55
Cereal		
	All-Bran Kellogs, 1/2 cup	42
	Bran Flakes, Post, 2/3 cup	74
	Cheerios, 1 cup	74
	Cocoa Krispies, 1 cup	77
	Corn Chex, 1 cup	83
	Corn Flakes, 1 cup	84
	Corn Pops, 1 cup	80
	Cream of Wheat, 1 oz.	74
	Frosted Flakes, 3/4 cup	55
	Froot Loops	69
	Grapenuts Flakes, 3/4 cup	80
	Frosted Mini Wheats, 1 cup	58
	Honey Smacks	71
	Multi Bran Chex, 1 cup	58
	Museli, 2/3 cup	43
	Raisin Bran, 3/4 cup	73
	Rice Chex, 1 1/4 cup	89
	Shredded Wheat, 1/2 cup	83
	Honey Smacks, 3/4 cup	56
	Special K, 1 cup	54
	Total, 3/4 cup	76
	Pancakes, from shake Mix	67
	Pop Tarts	70
Rice		

Category	Food Name	Glycemic Index
	Barley, pearled, 1/2 cup	25
	Couscous, 1/2 cup	65
	Instant, 1 cup, cooked	87
	Uncle Bens, converted, 1 cup	44
	Long grain White, 1 cup	41
	Short grain, white, 1 cup	72
	Rice Noodles	53
	Instant rice – white (boiled)	87
	Brown rice (boiled)	72
	Brown rice (steamed)	50
Cookies		
	Graham crackers	74
	Oatmeal cookie, 1 cookie	55
	Vanilla wafers, 7 cookies	77
Crackers		
	Rice cakes, plain, 3 cakes	82
	Stoned wheat thins, 3 crackers	67
	Water cracker, 3 crackers	78
Dairy		
	Ice cream, vanilla, 10% fat	61
	Low Fat Ice Cream	35
	Milk, whole, 1 cup	27
	Milk, skim, 1 cup	32
	Milk, chocolate, 1 cup, 1%	34
	Pudding, 1/2 cup	43
	Milk, soy, 1 cup	31
	Tofu frozen dessert, low fat, 1/2 cup	115
	Yogurt, nonfat, fruit, sugar, 8 oz.	33
	Yogurt, nonfat, plain, artificial sweet.	14
	Yogurt, nonfat, fruit, artificial sweet	14
	Custard, 3/4 cup	43
Fruits		

Category	Food Name	Glycemic Index
	Apple, 1 medium, 5 oz.	38
	Apple juice, unsweetened, 1 cup	40
	Apricots, 3 medium, 3 oz.	57
	Banana bread, 3 oz.	47
	Banana, 5 oz.	55
	Cherries, 10 large, 3 oz.	22
	Cranberry juice, 8 oz.	52
	Grapefruit, raw, 1/2 medium	25
	Grapes, green, 1 cup	46
	Kiwi, 1 medium	52
	Mango, 1 small	55
	Orange, 1 medium	44
	Orange juice, 1 cup	46
	Peach, 1 medium	30
	Pear, 1 medium	38
	Pineapple, 2 slices	66
	Plums, 1 medium	69
	Prunes, 6	29
	Raisins, 1/4 cup	64
	Watermelon, 1 cup	72
	Cantaloupe	65
Pasta / Pizza		
	Fettuccine, 6 oz.	45
	Linguine, 6 oz.	52
	Linguine with Shrimp Dinner	40
	Macaroni, 5 oz.	47
	Deluxe macaroni & Cheese Dinner	36
	Ravioli, meat, 4 large	39
	Ravioli, drum wheat flour, meat	39
	Spaghetti, white, 6 oz.	41
	Spaghetti, wheat, 6 oz.	37
	Spaghetti, white,	42

Category	Food Name	Glycemic Index
	boiled	
	Spiral, durum, 1 cup	43
	Tortellini, cheese, 8 oz.	50
	Vermicelli, 6 oz.	35
	Pizza, Super Supreme	36
	Pizza, Vegetarian Supreme (Pizza Hut)	49
	Lasagna, vegetarian	
	Lasagna, meat (Healthy Living brand)	20
	Lasagna, meat (Healthy Living brand)	28
	Lasagna, beef	47
Snacks		
	Vanilla wafers, 7 cookies	77
	Doughnut, deep-fried	75
	Apple Muffin	48
	Sponge cake, plain, 1 slice	46
	Snickers, 2.2 oz. Candy bar	41
	Pretzels, 1 oz.	83
	Potato chips, 14 pieces	54
	French Fries, 4.3 oz.	75
	Popcorn, light, microwave	55
	Popcorn, regular	72
	Pop Tarts, chocolate, 1 tart	70
	M&M's Chocolate candy, peanut	33
	Snickers Bar	41
	Mars Bar	68
	Peanuts	14
	Cashew nuts	25
	Granola Bar, chewy, 1 oz.	61
	Graham crackers, 4 squares	74
	Doritos Corn chips, 1 oz.	72
Drinks		
	Coca-Cola, 1 can, 12 oz.	77

Category	Food Name	Glycemic Index
	Gatorade, 8 oz.	78
	Fanta soft drink, 1 can, 12 oz.	63
	Apple Juice	40
	Orange Juice	50
	Tomato Juice	38
	Lemonade, sweetened	54
	Fruit Punch	67
	Chocolate Milk	34

Shopping / Food List

Smart Proteins

Chicken Breast / Skinless

Turkey Breast

Lean Ground Turkey

Top Round Steak

Top Sirloin Steak

Lean Ground Beef

Lean Ham

Lean Pork Chops

Lean Boneless Ribs

Wild Game Meats

Egg White

Egg Substitutes

Tune In Water

Swordfish

Steamed Haddock

Salmon Steamed

Crab / Lobster

Shrimp / Mussels

Low-Fat Cottage Cheese

Low-Fat Mozzarella

Tepheh / Seitan

Tofu

Vegetable Protein (T.V.P. Or Textured Vegetable Protein)

Soy Foods

Low Carb Jerky

Pure Protein Bars (Brand)

CARBmaster Yogurt (Kroger)

Buffalo

Wild Game

Turkey Bacon

Smart Carbs

Sweet Potatoes

Squash

Beans

Brown Rice

Wild Rice

Whole Grain Pasta

Veggie Pasta

Egg Noodles - Boiled

Oatmeal

High Fiber Cereal (i.e. Kashi Go Lean)

Whole Grain Tortillas

Whole Grain Breads (Ezekicl Is A Good Choice)

12 Grain Bread

Fruit (Any Kind)

Low Sugar Yogurt (i.e. Kroger brand CARBmaster yogurt)

Greek Yogurt

Whole Grain Bagels

Rice Cakes

Legumes

Beans (Any Kind)

Smart Vegetables

Broccoli

Asparagus

Lettuce

Carrots

Cauliflower

Green Beans

Bell Peppers

Mushrooms

Spinach

Tomatoes

V-8

Peas

Onions

Brussel Sprouts

Artichokes

Cabbage

Celery

Pickles

Zucchini

Cucumbers

Dark / Colored Salads

Hot Peppers

Leeks

Rhubarb

Smart Fats

Avocado

Sunflower Seeds

Pumpkin Seeds

Cold-Water Fish

Natural Peanut Butter

Dairy

Dressing / Condiments

Nuts

Olives

Olive Oil

Canola Oil

Sunflower Oil

Flax Seed Oil

Fish Oil

Fats To Avoid

Fried Foods

Hydrogenated Oils

Page Cycle Diet Daily Journal Page

Date:	Day of 90
Grams of protein:	
Ounces of water:	
Weight :	
Notes for the day: Emotional notes, etc.	

Selected Bibliography

"The Amazing Benefits of Nitric Oxide." Be Well Buzz. Halcyon Publishing, 06 Oct. 2010. Web. 15 Nov. 2011. <http://www.bewellbuzz. com/general/amazing-benefits-nitric-oxide/>.

Astrup, A., and S. Rossner. "Lessons from Obesity Management: Greater Initial Weight Loss Improves Long-term Maintenance." Obes Rev 1 (2000): 17-19. Print.

Astrup, A. "Prognostic markers for diet-induced weight loss in obese women." Int J Obes 9 (1995): 275-278

Astrup, Arne. "The Satiating Power of Protein—a Key to Obesity Prevention?" Am J Clin Nutr 82.1 (2005): 1-2. Print.

Botherston, Cindy. "Exercise Benefits. Learn the 60 Top Benefits of Exercise." Personal Trainer Cindy Brotherston for Fitness, Weight Loss and Nutrition. Web. Fall 2011. <http://www.busywomensfitness.com/exercise-benefits.html>.

"Dieting, Weight Loss & the Starvation Protection Mechanism." The Skinny on Weight Loss | Healthy Weight Loss Secrets. SuperSkinnyMe. com, 29 Oct. 2011. Web. 15 Nov. 2011. <http://www.superskinnyme.com/starvation_protection_mechanism.html>.

Doslon, Laura. "Insulin Resistance - What Is Insulin Resistance and How It Develops." Low Carb Diets at About.com - Atkins South Beach and More Low Carb Diets. About.com, 19 Sept. 2011. Web. 15 Nov. 2011. ⌐http://lowcarbdiets.about.com/od/prediabetesanddiabetes/a/insulinresistan.htm>.

Duse, Eleanor. "TLC Family "L-arginine: What You Need to Know""" Discovery Health "Health Guides" Web. Fall 2011. <http://health.howstuffworks.com/wellness/natural-medicine/alternative/l-arginine4.htm>.

Easdes, Michael R. "Metabolism and Ketosis." Web log post. The Blog of Michael R. Eades, M.D. 22 May 2007. Web. 15 Nov. 2011. <http://www.proteinpower.com/drmike/ketones-and-ketosis/metabolism-and-ketosis/>.

Elfhag, K. and Rossner, S. "Who succeeds in maintaining weight loss? A conceptual review of factors associated with weight loss maintenance and weight regain." Obes Rev 6 (2005): 67-85.

Fiore, Kristina. "Food Addiction Acts in Brain as Drug Addiction Does." Medical News and Free CME from MedPage Today. MedPage Today, 04 Apr. 2011. Web. 15 Nov. 2011. <http://www.medpagetoday.com/Psychiatry/Addictions/25713>.

Gilliatwimberly, M., M. Manore, K. Woolf, P. Swan, and S. Carroll. "Effects of Habitual Physical Activity on the Resting Metabolic Rates and Body Compositions of Women Aged 35 to 50 Years." Journal of the American Dietetic Association 101.10 (2001): 1181-188. Print.

Glycemic Index. Web. 15 Nov. 2011. <http://www.glycemicindex. com>.

"How Dieting And Age Affect Your Metabolism." How Dieting And Age Affect Your Metabolism. CalorieCount.About.com, 01 Jan. 2011. Web. 02 Jan. 2012. <http://caloriecount.about.com/article/how_dieting_and_age_affect_your_metabolism>.

InteSpringer Science+Business Media. "Shape up the quick way: Lose weight fast for lasting results suggests new study." ScienceDaily, 6 May 2010. Web. 15 Nov. 2011 < http://www.sciencedaily.com/releases/2010/05/100506092735.htm>

Joost, H.-G., and M. H. Tschop. "NO to Obesity: Does Nitric Oxide Regulate Fat Oxidation and Insulin Sensitivity?" Endocrinology 148.10 (2007): 4545-547. Print.

Lucotti, P., E. Setola, L. D. Monti, E. Galluccio, S. Costa, E. P. Sandoli, I. Fermo, G. Rabaiotti, R. Gatti, and P. Piatti. "Beneficial Effects of a Long-term Oral L-arginine Treatment Added to a Hypocaloric Diet and Exercise Training Program in Obese, Insulin-resistant Type 2 Diabetic Patients." AJP: Endocrinology and Metabolism 291.5 (2006): E906-912. Print.

Maki, Kevin C., Matthew S. Reeves, Mildred Farmer, Koichi Yasunaga, Noboru Matsuo, Yoshihisa Katsuragi, Masanori Komikado, Ichiro Tokimitsu, Donna Wilder, Franz Jones, Jeffrey B. Blumberg, and Yolanda Cartwright. "Green Tea Catechin Consumption Enhances Exercise-Induced Abdominal Fat Loss in Overweight and Obese Adults."

J. Nutr. 108.098293 (2008). Print. First published December 11, 2008, doi: 10.3945/jn.108.098293

McCARGAR, L., J. Sale, and S. M. Crawford. "Chronic Dieting Does Not Result in a Sustained Reduction in Resting Metabolic Rate in Overweight Women." Journal of the American Dietetic Association 96.11 (1996): 1175-177. Print.

Merimee, T. J., D. Rabinowitz, and S. E. Fineberg. "Arginine-Initiated Release of Human Growth Hormone — Factors Modifying the Response in Normal Man." N Engl J Med 280 (1969): 1434-438. Print.

Metzner, H. L., D. E. Lamphiear, N. C. Wheeler, and F. A. Larkin. "The Relationship between Frequency of Eating and Adiposity in Adult Men and Women in the Tecumseh Community Health Study." Am J Clin Nutr 30.5 (1977): 712-15. Print.

Nackers, L. M., K. M. Ross, and M. G. Perri. "The Association between Rate of Initial Weight Loss and Long-term Success in Obesity Treatment: Does Slow and Steady Win the Race?" International Journal of Behavioral Medicine 17.3 (2010): 161-67. Print.

Sniehotta, Falko F., Urte Scholz, Ralf Schwarzer, Bärbel Fuhrmann, Ulrich Kiwus, and Heinz Völler. "Long-term Effects of Two Psychological Interventions on Physical Exercise and Self-regulation following Coronary Rehabilitation." International Journal of Behavioral Medicine 12.4 (2005): 244-55. Print.

Study: Psychology Of Food Choices, What It Takes To Feel Truly

Satisfied. Pharmavite LLC. Pharmavite LLC, 16 Sept. 2009. Web. 15 Nov. 2011. <http://www.pharmavite.com/MediaCenter/MC_PR.asp?ID=166>.

"Theanine." Wikipedia, the Free Encyclopedia. Web. 15 Nov. 2011. <http://en.wikipedia.org/wiki/Theanine>.

Venables, Michelle C., Carl J. Hulston, Hannah R. Cox, and Asker E. Jeukendrup. "Green Tea Extract Ingestion, Fat Oxidation, and Glucose Tolerance in Healthy Humans." Am J Clin Nutr 87.3 (2008): 778-84. Print.

"Weight Training to Lose Weight?" Shelter Online. Shelter Publications, Inc., 2002. Web. Fall 2011. <http://www.shelterpub.com/_fitness/_office_fitness_clinic/OFC_wt_mgmt.html>.

Weigle, David S., Patricia A. Breen, Colleen C. Matthys, Holly S. Callahan, Kaatje E. Meeuws, Verna R. Burden, and Jonathan Q. Purnell. "A High-protein Diet Induces Sustained Reductions in Appetite, Ad Libitum Caloric Intake, and Body Weight despite Compensatory Changes in Diurnal Plasma Leptin and Ghrelin Concentrations." Am J Clin Nutr 82.1 (2005): 41-48. Print.

Acknowledgements

So many people had a hand in the book you are holding. I want to thank both Jennifers for taking my vision and making it a reality. Jennifer Du Charme, for the endless hours of dedication and hard work on the interior layout and content of the book. I could never have done it without her! Jennifer Phillips, for taking what I envisioned in my mind, and exceeding all expectations on the exterior layout of the book.

A special thanks to all of my clients, past and present, for believing in me and following my direction, no matter how crazy my ideas sound. Without your valuable feedback and willingness to give the "Page Cycle" 100%, the program would never be as powerful as it is today.

To my three boys, Braxton, Jordan, and Caden for always loving me and bringing so much happiness to my life. To Tracy, my sweetheart, for standing by me, through the tough times and for believing in me, even when I made poor choices.

Finally, and most of all, to my Dad who taught me how to work hard. Without his influence on my life, I would never have been able to get to the gym at 5:00am every day and put in 10 to 12 hours a day for twenty years. Even at 80 years old battling cancer, he never complains, and is still the hardest working man I know. I love you, Dad!

About The Author

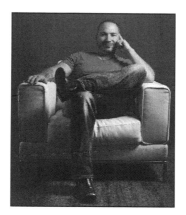

Mike Page graduated in 1991 from the University of Utah with a Bachelor's Degree in Exercise and Sports Science. He built the largest personal training businesses in Utah, at one point, employing over 60 trainers. Mike has performed over 50,000 individual personal training appointments, and has worked individually with over 4,000 clients. Three and a half years ago, Mike started working on a fast fat loss system called "The Page Cycle," that will be released in November 2011. Currently, over 30,000 people in over 32 countries are utilizing Mike's program with great success. The Page Cycle is a "Food Cycling" program that enables people to see instant results, combined with a long term plan to keep the weight off forever.

$$692$$
$$-100$$
$$592$$
$$320$$
$$272$$

$$320$$
$$100$$
$$692$$
$$420$$

$$272$$

$$432$$

$$692$$
$$-432$$
$$260$$

Made in the USA
Lexington, KY
23 April 2012